A Servier Service to Diabetes

DIABETES IN PRACTICE

DIABETES IN PRACTICE

Henry Connor
Consultant Physician, County Hospital, Hereford, UK

and

Andrew J M Boulton
Senior Lecturer in Medicine and Clinical Pharmacology,
University of Manchester,
and Consultant Physician,
Manchester Royal Infirmary, Manchester, UK

JOHN WILEY & SONS
Chichester · New York · Brisbane · Toronto · Singapore

Distributed in the United States of America, Canada
and Japan by Alan R. Liss Inc., 41 East 11th Street,
New York, NY 10003, USA.

Other Wiley Editorial Offices

John Wiley & Sons, Inc., 605 Third Avenue,
New York, NY 10158–0012, USA

Jacaranda Wiley Ltd, G.P.O. Box 859, Brisbane,
Queensland 4001, Australia

John Wiley & Sons (Canada) Ltd, 22 Worcester Road,
Rexdale, Ontario M9W 1L1, Canada

John Wiley & Sons (SEA) Pte Ltd, 37 Jalan Pemimpin   05-04
Block B, Union Industrial Building, Singapore 2057

Library of Congress Cataloging-in-Publication Data

Connor, H. (Henry)
      Diabetes in practice/Henry Connor and Andrew J.M. Boulton.
          p. cm.
      Includes bibliographies and index.
      ISBN 0 471 92087 8
      1. Diabetes — Treatment. I. Boulton, A.J.M. (Andrew James
Michael) II. Title.
      [DNLM: 1. Diabetes Mellitus. WK 810 C752d]
      RC660.C66   1989
      616.4′62 — dc20
      DNLM/DLC
      for Library of Congress

British Library Cataloguing in Publication Data
Connor, H. (Henry)
   Diabetes in practice.
   1. Man. Diabetes. Therapy
   I. Title II. Boulton, A.J.M. (Andrew James
Michael)
   616.4′6206

   ISBN 0 471 92087 8

Printed in Great Britain at the Alden Press
Oxford London and Northampton

CONTENTS

FOREWORD

R.D. Lawrence began the Preface to the first edition of *The Diabetic Life* in 1925 by stating that the object of his book was to bring the modern treatment of diabetes within the scope of the busy general practitioner. It must be stated, almost 50 years later, that community care for patients with diabetes is increasing. Most general practitioners are involved with some aspects of diabetes care, either being responsible for diabetes care *per se* or looking after other clinical problems in patients with diabetes. The last 15 years have seen the evolution of many different diabetes management schemes. These range from hospital-based clinic care at one end of the spectrum to total general practice care at the other. It is probably a minority of patients who need total hospital care but most patients will benefit from the occasional visit to the local consultant.

I consider the development of shared care schemes to be one of the most exciting and progressive areas of diabetes management taking place at present. These schemes combine the expertise of the consultant diabetes specialist with the general practitioner's detailed knowledge of the patient's general health and social situation. Successful diabetes management now depends on a co-ordinated team approach involving the patients, parents and relatives, a specialist nurse, the practice nurse, dietitian, chiropodist, general practitioner and a consultant, and includes a great deal of patient education. It has been quite conclusively shown that the patient's attitude to diabetes management can influence metabolic control.

There are tremendous benefits in becoming closely involved with diabetic patients and enormous potential within general practice to improve their care without having to rely heavily on the hospital service. However, in order for this step to be taken, it is vitally important that accurate up-to-date easily readable information is available in order for members of the primary health care team to be fully informed. Drs Henry Connor and Andrew Boulton have been remarkably successful in completing this task. The content of 'Diabetes in Practice' is extremely accessible and well laid out, covering all the aspects of diabetes care that busy general practitioners and their extended team, especially the practice nurse, need to know in order to benefit their patients.

P.R.W. TASKER
Principal in General Practice
St James's House Surgery,
County Court Road,
Kings Lynn, Norfolk, PE30 5EJ

PREFACE

The provision of diabetes care by general practitioners has increased greatly in the last few years, but until now there has been no book intended primarily for those general practitioners and practice nurses who wish to be involved in the management of their diabetic patients. We hope that this book will fill that gap. We are extremely grateful to Dr Peter Tasker, a general practitioner with special experience in diabetes, who has read the entire manuscript, for his very helpful comments and for contributing the Foreword. We also wish to thank the many other colleagues, both general practitioners and hospital doctors, for their suggestions. Any errors are, of course, our own responsibility. We are extremely grateful to our secretaries, Mrs Pat Rossi and Ms Anne Timms, for typing the manuscript and for incorporating all our amendments and afterthoughts with such good grace; and finally, we would like to thank the medical and administrative personnel at Servier Laboratorires, without whose financial support and help this venture would not have been possible.

H. CONNOR
A.J.M. BOULTON

ABBREVIATIONS

BDA	British Diabetic Association
CSII	Continuous Subcutaneous Insulin Infusion
DKA	Diabetic Ketoacidosis
ESRD	End Stage Renal Disease
FBG	Fasting Blood Glucose
GDM	Gestational Diabetes Mellitus
$HbA_1 C$/GlyHb	Glycosylated Haemoglobin
HBGM	Home Blood Glucose Monitoring
HLA	Human Leucocyte Antigen
IGT	Impaired Glucose Tolerance
MSU	Mid-Stream Urine
OHG	Oral Hypoglycaemic Drug
OGTT	Oral Glucose Tolerance Test
PVD	Peripheral Vascular Disease
RBG	Random Blood Glucose
RCGP	Royal College of General Practitioners
Type I Diabetes IDDM	Insulin Dependent Diabetes Mellitus (former terms: juvenile onset, ketosis-prone)
Type II Diabetes NIDDM	Non-Insulin Dependent Diabetes Mellitus (former terms: late onset, maturity onset, non-ketosis prone)
VLCD	Very Low Calorie Diet
WHO	World Health Organization

1 WHY CARE FOR DIABETIC PATIENTS IN GENERAL PRACTICE?

A simple answer to this question is that half the patients are not attending a hospital clinic and are already dependent on their general practitioner for all aspects of diabetes management. There are, however, more positive reasons why general practitioners might wish to consider providing an organised system of care for their diabetic patients.

1. Successful management requires the co-operation of the patient and his family. The general practitioner's knowledge of the patient, his family and the home circumstances makes it easier to set realistic targets for the patient.
2. A diagnosis of diabetes means follow-up for life, and the general practitioner is usually better placed than a hospital doctor to provide continuity of care.
3. Much of diabetes management is preventative medicine which is primarily the province of primary health care teams.
4. The general practitioner is a family doctor and diabetes is a disorder which affects the whole family. If the patient has to eat at a particular time of day it is likely that the rest of the family will have to do so too, and, like it or not, they will probably have to eat the same food which the patient has been advised to eat. Any member of the family may have to deal with hypoglycaemia or other diabetes problems.
5. For most patients a visit to the general practitioner's surgery is more convenient and less costly than an appointment at the hospital clinic.

Diabetes care offers the practitioner a combination of preventative medicine, acute medical care and family medicine. Done well it is interesting and rewarding.

2 ORGANISING DIABETES CARE IN GENERAL PRACTICE

Following the introduction of insulin into clinical practice, many hospitals set up specialist clinics for diabetes care and by the early 1950s most district general hospitals had a diabetic clinic. These clinics provided a focal point for diabetes management, and for many years it was tacitly assumed that the needs of all diabetic patients were best provided for in a hospital clinic. In fact about half of all diabetic patients were not attending a hospital clinic, either because they had never been referred or because the patients themselves found the clinics unsatisfactory in one way or another. Half of the diabetic population was not therefore receiving any organised form of medical care. Only in the last 10 to 15 years has serious consideration been given to the idea that general practitioners could provide the service which these patients need, and that many of the patients who were attending hospital clinics could be looked after just as well, or even better, by their own doctors.

If we consider the evolving pattern of obstetric care during this century we find an interesting contrast with diabetes management. Obstetrics was traditionally a matter for the general practitioner. Most antenatal care was provided by him and most deliveries took place in the patients' own homes. Only when major problems arose were the patients referred to hospital. Over the years, however, a well-organised system of shared care provided by both general practitioner and consultant has evolved. There are three lessons to be learned from the obstetric experience:

1. Shared care can work, and does work, to the mutual benefit of all concerned.
2. Organisation is the key to success.
3. An annual assessment of maternal and perinatal mortality has resulted in improved standards of health care.

In the management of diabetes these are lessons which both hospital doctors and general practitioners are only just beginning to learn and to apply.

■ Essential prerequisites for successful diabetes care

1. An organised system of care

An organised system for the delivery of diabetes care is essential. Without such a system regular follow-up becomes uncertain, blood glucose concentrations are not checked and eyes are not examined. This has been shown in several studies. The initiation and maintenance of organised diabetes care requires the combined efforts of an interested and enthusiastic general practitioner, a practice nurse or health visitor and the practice secretary or clerk.

2. A diabetic register and recall system

The practice of preventative medicine requires that all diabetic patients be identified and that they be seen at predetermined intervals, with a method for identifying and recalling those who default.

The register can be compiled from personal knowledge and by checks on repeat prescriptions. These simple methods will identify the great majority of patients within a few months because most patients test their urine or blood for glucose, even if they do not require oral hypoglycaemics or insulin.

Those practices which have a computer may wish to use it for both the register and the recall system, but simpler devices are just as effective. The simplest is a card index in a small box. Each patient is given a card and the box also contains 12 divider cards, one for each month of the year. If a patient is seen in January and asked to return in July his card is then placed in the July slot. At the end of each month the practice secretary checks for any cards that still remain in the current month's section. In this way defaulters are easily identified and can be recalled.

3. Diabetic records

A specialised record card is essential. The design should be such that any known diabetic complications are prominently displayed and it should be easy to see when the next annual review is due. Results of measurements such as body weight, blood glucose or visual acuity should be in columns so that any change is readily apparent. Examples of suitable record cards can be found in the RCGP *Diabetes* folder, and several pharmaceutical companies also provide record cards which fit into the FP 5/6 envelopes still used by most general practitioners. When a patient's care is shared between the general practitioner and a hospital clinic it may be more convenient to allow the patient to keep the record, in the same way as antenatal patients keep their shared-care cards. The patient's general notes should be marked with a diabetes label. Brown is the RCGP colour-code for diabetes.

4. Access to other services

i. *Laboratory services*
    Access to measurements of blood glucose, glycosylated haemoglobin, renal function and serum lipids is essential.

ii. *Dietetic advice*
    Ideally all diabetic patients should be advised by a dietitian (see Chapter 4).

iii. *Chiropody*
    Chiropody is an essential preventative measure for many patients (see Chapter 8).

iv. *Ophthalmological expertise*
    Annual screening for the detection of early retinopathy is mandatory (Chapter 8). Whether the screening is done by the general practitioner himself, an ophthalmic optician or a hospital doctor will depend on the expertise of the general practitioner and on local arrangements for retinopathy screening. It is the responsibility of the doctor who takes overall care for the patient's diabetes to make sure that someone examines the eyes, if he himself does not. If retinopathy is discovered the indications for referral to an ophthalmologist are described in Chapter 8.

5. Literature for patients

All patients should be given the following items.

- **Simple educational literature** to re-inforce what they have been told verbally.

- **A record book** in which to keep details of urine or blood glucose tests, hypoglycaemic attacks and details of dosages of insulin or hypoglycaemics.

- **An identity card** if they are treated with oral hypoglycaemics or insulin.

Suitable literature can be obtained from the hospital diabetes clinic, the British Diabetic Association and from a number of pharmaceutical companies who manufacture insulin or oral hypoglycaemic drugs (Appendix 5). There are obvious advantages in using the same record books and literature as are provided by the diabetes clinic at the local hospital.

One or more doctors?

In some practices there will be just one general practitioner who takes a specialist interest in diabetes management. In others the partners consider that they should all be involved to preserve continuity of care for their own patients. Each system has its advantages and disadvantages. If one doctor sees all the diabetic patients he develops a greater expertise but that expertise is not available when he is on holiday. If all the doctors participate then the patient can see his own family doctor but the individual partners have less experience of diabetes management. The choice must be made by each practice. If more than one doctor participates the organisation of follow-up becomes more complicated but this is not an insuperable problem.

Specialist mini-clinics — essential or unnecessary?

Most of the general practitioners who offer an organised system of diabetes care have instituted diabetic mini-clinics, but others have thought such clinics unnecessary and see their diabetic patients during the course of ordinary surgeries.

Mini-clinics do have some definite advantages:

1. The clinic can be organised so that adequate time is allowed for each patient. This subject is discussed in more detail below.
2. Involvement of the practice nurse can be ensured, and it is easier to ensure that weighing, urine testing, etc., are carried out.
3. The organisation of follow-up appointments and the detection of defaulters is simplified.
4. A mini-clinic helps to create the right frame of mind for 'thinking diabetic'.
5. A mini-clinic makes it feasible for the community dietitian or local diabetologist to attend, if and when required.

On the other hand, some would argue that a mini-clinic creates a 'production-line approach'. However this need not be a problem if the clinic is properly organised. Attendance during normal surgery hours can be more convenient for patients because it allows them flexibility in the times at which they can attend. If patients are to be seen in normal surgeries then some means of offering them 'protected time' is essential. **An adequate annual review requires 20–30 minutes** and cannot be compressed into the seven or eight minutes available during a normal surgery appointment. A large part of the annual review can, of course, be done by a practice nurse who has had appropriate training.

It is our view that the needs of the diabetic patient are best served by a combination of mini-clinic and ordinary surgery visits. One or possibly two visits a year to a mini-clinic will provide adequate time for a detailed review of the diabetes, in a context where the skills of doctor and practice nurse can be combined, and in a system which ensures continuity of regular follow-up and detection of defaulters. Problems which arise between these review visits can be dealt with at visits during normal surgery hours. For example, if the dose of oral hypoglycaemic is altered at a review clinic, the patient can come to an ordinary surgery two months later to check that the desired effect has been achieved.

How much of a doctor's time does a specialist mini-clinic require?

A practice with four partners and a list size of 9000 will have about 108 diabetic patients on its books (assuming a prevalence rate for diabetes of 1.2%). If we also assume that two-thirds of these patients are under the sole care of their general practitioner there will be 72 patients requiring mini-clinic visits for an annual review. Allowing 30 minutes for each review gives a total of 36 hours p.a., equivalent to a three hour clinic once a month. Some of this time would in any case be required during ordinary surgery visits if there were no mini-clinics, so the extra workload is not particularly burdensome.

■ The role of the practice nurse

The services of a practice nurse are a major advantage in the delivery of diabetes health care. Patients and their relatives will sometimes confide in and seek advice from the nurse rather than 'bothering the doctor'. Depending on local arrangements within the district for education of the diabetic patient (see Chapter 9), the nurse may be required to provide some or all of the patient's diabetes education. If she is to teach more than basic urine testing techniques or simple foot care advice then the practice should consider funding her to take the English National Board course in Diabetic

Nursing (ENB No. 928 — see Appendix 5 for address). The nurse can help at the review clinic by measuring weight and blood pressure, checking urine samples and visual acuity and, in some practices, examining the feet and taking blood samples. A successful nurse can become the focal point for diabetes care in the practice, especially if more than one doctor is involved in diabetes management. She can make arrangements for referrals to the chiropodist and dietitian and liaise with the hospital diabetes service through the district nurse-specialist in diabetes.

■ Who should be referred for hospital follow-up?

The answer to this question will depend in part on the expertise which is available in the practice. For example, a general practitioner with particular experience of diabetes management may be able to look after patients whom another doctor would be best advised to refer.

When considering which patients are suitable for general practice care it is important to dispel the myth of 'mild diabetes'. **There is no such condition as 'mild diabetes'**. The need for insulin treatment is not a measure of the severity of the diabetes. There are patients who are treated with diet alone and whose diabetic control is apparently excellent, but who still develop sight-threatening retinopathy or neuropathic and vascular complications which result in amputation. **Apparently good control in a patient who requires only a simple diet is not a cause for complacency**. Unless the general practitioner can offer an organised system of care, as described in the preceding pages, even these patients should be considered for referral to a hospital clinic.

Patients who should normally be referred to a hospital clinic

1. *Children, adolescent and pregnant diabetic patients*
   Few general practitioners have the expertise to manage the special problems posed by these patients.

2. *Patients whose control is not good*
   The question of what constitutes good diabetic control is discussed in Chapter 6. Any patient whose control is thought to be inadequate deserves a second opinion, even if it is thought that the reason for the poor control lies primarily in the patient's hands.

3. *Patients with diabetic complications*
Most of these patients should be reviewed by a consultant, even if they are seen only once to confirm that the current management is correct or to suggest guidelines for further treatment.

Further reading

Day J.L., Humphreys H. and Alban-Davies H. (1987). Problems of comprehensive shared diabetes care. *British Medical Journal* **294**, 1590–1592.

Gibbins R.L., Rowlands C.J. and Saunders J. (1986). A management system for diabetes in general practice. *Diabetic Medicine* **3**, 477–479.

Graham M.A.H. (1986). Starting a diabetic clinic. *Practical Diabetes* **3**(3), 135–136.

Hill R.D. *Diabetes Health Care*. Chapman and Hall, London, 1987, chapters 6 and 13.

Irving J.M.R., Casement S.M. and Holme Q. (1988). A 'no-clinic' system of care for non-insulin-dependent diabetics in general practice. *Practical Diabetes* **5**(3), 125–128.

RCGP. *Diabetes* (a folder containing a collection of articles, pamphlets and information). The Library and Information Service of The Royal College of General Practitioners, London, 1986.

Tasker P.R.W. (1984). Is diabetes a disease for general practice? *Practical Diabetes* **1**(1), 21–24.

Waine C. *Why Not Care for Your Diabetic Patients?* The Royal College of General Practitioners, London, 1986, 42 pp.

3 WHAT IS DIABETES?

Diabetes mellitus may be defined as a chronic metabolic disorder that is characterised by elevation of the blood glucose concentration and caused by a relative or absolute deficiency of insulin. This simple definition encompasses the two main types of primary diabetes and in addition the many, though much rarer, causes of secondary diabetes. Diabetes not only causes profound abnormalities of carbohydrate metabolism, but also affects protein and fat metabolism leading to a catabolic state. If left untreated, diabetes will ultimately lead to a state that may be best described as 'metabolic chaos'.

■ Establishing the diagnosis

The diagnosis of diabetes must always be made by measuring blood glucose and demonstrating its unequivocal elevation. A full oral glucose tolerance test (OGTT) is rarely required to make the diagnosis, and is often performed unnecessarily in patients with symptoms and elevated random blood glucose levels (Table 1). This test is expensive both in terms of the laboratory and the patient's time. **Glycosuria** alone is suggestive, but not diagnostic of diabetes. **Glycosuria and ketonuria** in a young person with classic symptoms is almost certainly indicative of diabetes, but demonstration of an elevated blood glucose level is still required to make the diagnosis.

The WHO criteria for diabetes state that a result of greater than 8 mmol/l (fasting) or 11 mmol/l (random) confirms the diagnosis. **It must be noted that these readings are for venous plasma**: if venous or capillary whole blood is analysed, the values are slightly lower. The method of analysis should be printed on the chemical pathology laboratory result form. As the diagnosis of diabetes has serious implications, the patient should be asked to return for a repeat fasting blood glucose test if the result is borderline.

TABLE 1 DIAGNOSTIC CRITERIA FOR DIABETES (NON-PREGNANT)

	Venous plasma glucose (mmol/l)		
	Normal	Impaired glucose tolerance	Diabetes
Fasting	< 6	> 6	> 8
Two hours after 75 g glucose load	< 8	> 8 < 11	> 11

Note: Based on WHO recommendations. Values for whole blood or capillary samples will be slightly lower.

It is only in those cases where doubt remains that an OGTT may be needed. A number of older terms such as 'latent' or 'chemical' diabetes are no longer used: an individual now has frank diabetes, normal glucose tolerance, or impaired glucose tolerance (IGT) if results are equivocal (see Table 1).

The definition of IGT was introduced after several epidemiological studies demonstrated that subjects with blood glucose values within this range (Table 1) are more prone to develop macrovascular disease although they rarely develop other specific long-term diabetic complications. There is no general concensus as to how patients with IGT should be managed, but weight reduction, if appropriate, and treatment of any associated hyperlipidaemia are advisable in younger patients with this condition.

The above definitions all refer to non-pregnant individuals. **Gestational diabetes** (GDM) is defined as diabetes which develops during pregnancy and later remits (see also Chapter 11). The criteria for the diagnosis of GDM are different: fasting blood glucose (venous plasma) > 5.8 mmol/l and/or if any other reading during a 75 g OGTT is > 8 mmol/l. Those diagnosed as having GDM need to be managed as if they had frank diabetes, with diligent follow-up and monitoring: such patients should be referred to the hospital clinic and many hospitals run a joint obstetric/diabetes clinic. Those women who are at greater risk of developing GDM are listed in Table 2.

■ Types of diabetes

Primary diabetes includes the two main types for which the immediate cause is not apparent. Type I or insulin-dependent diabetes accounts for approximately 10% of primary diabetes whereas Type II or non-insulin

TABLE 2 RISK FACTORS FOR GESTATIONAL DIABETES

- Strong family history of diabetes
- Fasting glycosuria
- Previous unexplained perinatal loss
- Previous 'large for dates' infant
- Previous gestational diabetes
- Gross maternal obesity

dependent diabetes accounts for 90%. Cases of secondary diabetes (where an underlying cause is readily apparent) are rare.

Type I diabetes

The term Type I diabetes was adopted to replace the older terminology such as 'juvenile-onset' diabetes as the condition may occur at any age, though it most commonly presents in those less than 30 years old. Patients with Type I diabetes are usually severely insulinopaenic, ketosis-prone and are dependent on exogenous insulin for life. The prevalence of this condition amongst school children in the UK is about 0.2% and rising, and it affects both sexes approximately equally. Both genetic and environmental factors contribute to its aetiology. Although Type I diabetes is more common in individuals with certain HLA types, there is no clear pattern of inheritance and only half of the monozygotic twins of Type I diabetes patients develop the disease. If one parent has the condition, the risk of a child developing Type I diabetes, though increased, is still only about 1–4%. It is thought that certain environmental factors — such as a viral infection — may precipitate the onset of diabetes in a genetically prone individual. There is now known to be a long 'pre-diabetic' period during which there is an 'auto-immune' attack on the pancreatic islet cells. Clinical diabetes usually presents when about 90% of the insulin producing beta cells have been destroyed.

Future research may enable potential diabetic subjects to be identified before the clinical disease presents so that intervention might prevent the disease developing. At present, double-blind trials of Cyclosporin are in progress to see if this might enable the 10% of functioning islets to be saved at the time of clinical diagnosis.

Clinical presentation
The diagnosis of Type I diabetes rarely presents a clinical challenge: the patient is usually young and complains of the classical symptoms as listed in Table 3. The presentation is often acute with symptoms of a few weeks'

TABLE 3 SYMPTOMS SUGGESTIVE OF DIABETES

- Thirst
- Polyuria, nocturia
- Weight loss
- Pruritus vulvae, balanitis
- Blurred vision
- Lethargy

duration in a patient with a history of recent weight loss. Blurring of vision, due to osmotic changes in the lens, and non-specific symptoms such as tiredness and lethargy are common. It must also be remembered that Type I diabetes may present as an acute emergency such as diabetic ketoacidosis (DKA). A viral or bacterial illness may precipitate DKA in a patient with little islet cell reserve.

> Thus, any patient with a history suggestive of diabetes requires **urgent** urinalysis for glucose and ketones, together with a random blood glucose reading which, in the first instance, should be done in the surgery using either a meter or a blood glucose strip (Glucostix or BM sticks). Any patient showing heavy glycosuria and ketonuria, together with marked elevation of blood glucose needs immediate hospital referral by telephone.

Type II diabetes

Although Type II diabetes may present at any age (hence the term 'maturity-onset' is no longer used), it typically occurs in patients over 45 years old. Its overall prevalence in the UK is approximately 1%, but this rises to 5% in subjects older than 75. Unlike Type I diabetes, it is much more common in women, and obesity, pregnancy and parity are all potential contributory factors to its aetiology. Hereditary factors are stronger in Type II diabetes: the monozygotic twins of Type II diabetic patients almost always develop diabetes themselves, although there may be a delay of several years before symptoms develop in the co-twin. The main environmental factor in the aetiology of Type II diabetes is food: diabetes is commoner in the obese, although only a minority of obese people develop Type II diabetes. Thus, as in Type I diabetes, a combination of genetic and environmental factors probably causes the disease. Another relevant environmental factor that warrants mention is stress: many patients report that the diagnosis of diabetes was made following a stressful event such as an accident or a bereavement. The most likely explanation is that the stress precipitated or unmasked the diabetes in a patient who would eventually have developed the disease.

A number of defects may lead to the development of Type II diabetes:

1. reduced insulin secretion by the beta cells,
2. altered hepatic handling of glucose,
3. insulin resistance at the cellular level.

Thus the aetiology of diabetes may be described as being heterogenous.

Clinical presentation
The diagnosis of Type II diabetes may be more difficult as the clinical presentation can be extremely variable. Patients often present with some of the symptoms listed in Table 3 though the symptoms tend to be milder and of longer duration. Weight loss is less common whereas pruritus vulvae or balanitis are more frequently problematic. However, many patients have no symptoms whatsoever and are found to have diabetes at a routine medical or insurance examination. A third group of patients present with complications of their diabetes as they may well have had asymptomatic hyperglycaemia for many years. Thus any older patient who develops neuropathy, unexplained foot ulceration or visual disturbance should be screened for diabetes.

Secondary diabetes

Diabetes may occasionally develop as a consequence of other disease or drug therapy and a summary of some of these causes is provided in Table 4. A high index of suspicion should be maintained when patients develop these conditions, or, for example, are treated with steroids.

TABLE 4 SOME CAUSES OF SECONDARY DIABETES

- Pancreatic disease
  (pancreatitis, surgery, carcinoma, cystic fibrosis)
- Endocrine diseases
  (e.g. acromegaly, Cushings)
- Drugs
  (e.g. steroids, contraceptive pill, diuretics)
- Genetic syndromes
  (many described — all extremely rare)

■ Consequences of untreated diabetes

The clinical consequences or natural history of untreated diabetes depend
on the type of diabetes. Nowadays we can only fully appreciate the consequences of untreated Type I diabetes by reading the horrific reports of the
fate of insulin-dependent patients in the pre-insulin era (see Further
reading). However, the diagnosis of Type I diabetes may still be missed
because of an unusual presentation. Those patients whose main symptom
is fatigue or lethargy may be initially prescribed an anti-depressant; severe
weight loss may be ascribed to anorexia, and nocturia or enuresis may
prompt a renal referral. Untreated Type I diabetes invariably leads to
metabolic decompensation and the development of ketoacidosis. Prior to
1922, patients died either of overwhelming infection or DKA. However, a
recent survey of deaths in diabetic patients under the age of 50 showed that
patients are still dying in DKA. As this is a preventable problem, **death
should never be a consequence**: in the ill diabetic patient, the urine
should be tested for glucose and ketones, and should any doubt about the
diagnosis remain, immediate referral to hospital is indicated.

Type II patients are not ketosis prone and may have asymptomatic
hyperglycaemia for years before diabetes is diagnosed. However, some
patients are difficult to classify as Type I or Type II as they may have
features of both conditions. It is important to ask the question 'Is insulin
therapy indicated in this patient?' if any doubt exists. In general, those thin
patients with pronounced symptoms of rapid onset warrant insulin therapy
whatever age they may be, though further discussion and guidelines are to
be found in Chapter 5.

It is generally accepted that the long-term complications of diabetes are
related to preceding glycaemic control and the duration of the condition.
However, as some patients have no evidence of any complications after
many years of hyperglycaemia whereas, conversely, some patients develop
severe complications after a few years of apparently good control, there can
be little doubt that there is, in addition, a genetic predisposition to certain
of the diabetes related complications. Recent evidence, for example,
suggests that patients with nephropathy frequently have a family history of
hypertension, suggesting a possible genetic association. It is, therefore,
unwise to label a patient as having 'mild' diabetes: such a patient with mild
hyperglycaemia may still have severe microvascular complications, peripheral vascular disease and impotence. It is to be hoped that clinical research
will eventually enable us to recognise, at diagnosis, which patients are more
prone to later complications, so that efforts to achieve normoglycaemia
could be concentrated on such individuals.

■ Aims and principles of management

The aims and principles of management have not changed since Dr R.D. Lawrence, the famous diabetologist, founding member of the British Diabetic Association and himself a diabetic, summarized them as 'education and understanding about diabetes and aiming to lead a normal life'. Thus, in summary, the aims of any treatment plan should be to relieve symptoms, and to avoid both short and long-term complications with minimal interference of day-to-day life.

Diabetes is almost unique amongst chronic medical conditions in that there is no cure, it has lifelong consequences, and the patients and their families need to have a thorough understanding of the condition and its consequences. The patients themselves make many important decisions about their care, and appropriate judgement and action at home may ultimately prevent a minor problem from becoming a major one. Thus the principles of management may be summarized under the following headings.

Patient understanding

Successful management of diabetes requires the active participation of the patient and education must therefore start at diagnosis and continue thereafter. Although this is discussed in detail in Chapter 9, education must include an understanding of diabetes and of the treatments used, the acute and possible long-term complications and how to assess the level of control. The provision of leaflets and booklets alone is insufficient: each consultation should be used as an educational exercise in addition to the assessment of medical problems and prescribing of appropriate therapy.

Dietary principles

All diabetic patients require dietary advice, which may vary from a simple weight-reducing high-fibre diet for a newly-diagnosed obese Type II diabetic patient to the complex diet for a Type I patient who works shifts and has established renal disease requiring sodium and protein restrictions. In addition, most patients should be encouraged to take more exercise (see also Chapter 4).

Oral hypoglycaemic agents and insulin

All patients with Type I diabetes require insulin treatment in addition to dietary modifications. Conversely, some patients with Type II diabetes can be managed satisfactorily on diet alone, though the majority will ultimately require the addition of OHGs or insulin (see also Chapter 5).

Lifestyle adjustments

The diagnosis of diabetes may have a major impact on an individual's lifestyle (Chapter 10). This may include a change in occupation (e.g. airline pilot), increases in insurance premiums, reduction of alcohol intake and advice to stop smoking. One advantage is the exemption from prescription charges for those treated with OHGs or insulin.

The diagnosis of diabetes may have profound implications for the patient: a compassionate and reassuring approach is required. Essential information should be given when the diagnosis is first made, with reinforcement and further education being provided at subsequent visits. The necessary information for patient management and education is provided in the remaining chapters.

■ Further reading

Bliss M. (1982). *The Discovery of Insulin*. Paul Harris Publishing Co., p. 6.

4 DIET AND DIABETES

■ Diet as a cause of diabetes

Excessive consumption of dietary energy results in obesity which is a major risk factor for Type II (non-insulin dependent) diabetes. The nature of the food which is eaten has also been implicated in the causation of Type II diabetes. For example, diabetes is common in recently urbanised populations and this observation can be linked to consumption of an increased quantity of refined carbohydrate with a reduction in the amount of carbohydrate which is unrefined and associated with its natural complement of fibre.

There is no convincing evidence that diet is implicated in the pathogenesis of Type I (insulin dependent) diabetes.

■ Diet in the management of diabetes

Diet is the foundation stone of diabetic treatment, and for many patients it is the only treatment which is needed. Those who also require oral hypoglycaemics or insulin are unlikely to maintain good control of their diabetes unless they also observe certain dietary principles.

Dietary recommendations have altered considerably in recent years. The low carbohydrate–high fat diets which were a relic of the pre-insulin era are obsolete.

The principles of modern dietary management are:

1. The avoidance or correction of obesity by limitation of energy (calorie) intake where appropriate.
2. An increase in the consumption of dietary energy from unrefined (high fibre) carbohydrate, so that total carbohydrate intake accounts for at least 50% of dietary energy.

---

3. A reduction in consumption of fats so that energy from these sources accounts for less than 35%, and ideally about 30%, of total energy intake. Saturated fat should account for 10% or less of total energy intake.
4. Food intake should be evenly distributed throughout the day, and the distribution should remain reasonably consistent from day to day.

Putting theory into practice

Although the first three principles are identical to those which are now recommended for the general population, they do represent a significant change from the typical 'western' diet (Table 1). We are therefore asking many of our patients to make radical alterations in their eating habits. These changes will not only affect the patient but may also involve other members of the family, because it is not usually practical to prepare separate meals. We must therefore be prepared to meet with some resistance, and changes may have to be introduced gradually. For example, we cannot reasonably expect a patient who is used to eating only ten grams of fibre daily to double or treble this intake overnight. This would represent a major social change and might well cause abdominal discomfort or pain, so we should not therefore be surprised if the patient ignored our advice.

Expert advice and tuition from a trained dietitian is essential for the great majority of diabetic patients. Dietitians have the knowledge and expertise to tailor diets to suit individual preferences and foibles which

TABLE 1 RECOMMENDED AND ACTUAL SOURCES OF DIETARY ENERGY

Energy source	Per cent of dietary energy	
	Recommended diet	Typical diet
Carbohydrate	> 50	40–45
Protein	15	15
Fat	c. 30	40–45

Note: The recommendations are based on those of the Diabetes and Nutrition Study Group of the European Association for the Study of Diabetes (1988).

makes life much more tolerable for the patient and improves compliance. Without such help the patient is likely to eat a rather limited range of foods and will soon get bored with the whole business, reverting to former eating habits. Dietitians are better able than doctors to answer patients' questions. If you have to refer to a book to answer simple questions about the carbohydrate content of different foods (and most doctors do) the patient may start to think that diet cannot be all that important. Your role as the doctor is to determine the type of diet which is appropriate for the individual patient, and the dietitian's role is to put the dietary prescription into practice. (If you do not have access to a dietitian you will need to learn more about dietary management than is contained in this book. This problem is discussed later in the chapter.)

Stop-gap advice while waiting to see the dietitian

Newly diagnosed patients need some interim advice while waiting for their appointment with the dietitian. The British Diabetic Association (see Appendix 5 for address) has produced a leaflet entitled *Food and Diabetes — just a beginning* which is intended for just this purpose and every surgery should keep a supply. As a stop-gap measure this leaflet is preferable to the more detailed diet sheets distributed by some pharmaceutical companies because advice contained in these may conflict with that in the definitive diet given by the dietitian, and this inevitably causes confusion.

The diet prescription — what the dietitian needs to know

'Diabetic diet, please' is a common form of referral to the dietitian, but if she is to give your patient the correct advice the dietitian needs rather more information. For example, if the patient is overweight you will want to reduce his consumption of calories. For an office worker a standard '1000 calorie high fibre' diet may well be appropriate, but this would be totally inappropriate for someone engaged in heavy manual work. In such a case you may leave the dietitian to decide on a suitable number of calories, but if you want to specify how stringent the diet should be your diet prescription might read 'Please assess present calorie intake and reduce it by 40%'. If a target weight has been agreed with the patient, it will help the dietitian to know this. An appropriate target weight might be the average weight for height and age (see Appendix 1), but if this seems unrealistic in a very obese patient then a compromise should be agreed with the patient. If you want the energy intake to be distributed in a particular fashion then say so. It may also be helpful to give your opinion of what it is reasonable to expect of the patient. For example, if you know that the patient is illiterate do tell the dietitian! If it is the patient's wife who prepares all the meals then ask the patient to take his wife with him when he sees the dietitian.

Carbohydrate portions or exchanges

Some patients, especially those treated with insulin, need a means of ensuring that they eat approximately the same amount of carbohydrate at the same time each day. This can be achieved by use of the 'portion' or 'exchange' system. A portion or exchange is defined as the amount of food which contains 10 grams of carbohydrate. (The British Diabetic Association publishes tables of the carbohydrate content of all the common foods.) For example, an apple contains approximately 10 grams of carbohydrate and therefore constitutes one portion, as does one digestive or wholemeal biscuit. By referring to the published tables a patient who has a mid-morning snack of 10 grams (one portion) of carbohydrate might decide to eat an apple one day, and on the next day to exchange the apple for a large digestive or wholemeal biscuit.

Examples of typical diet prescriptions are shown in the boxes below.

Patient A

An estate agent, aged 59, who is 20 kg above the average weight for height and age and has a serum cholesterol concentration of 7.2 mmol/l.

Prescription: '1000 calorie diet, encourage increased consumption of fibre, reduce refined carbohydrate and fat. Maximum of one alcoholic drink per day, to be included in calorie allowance. No target weight set, let's see how he gets on. A bon viveur! No drug therapy.'

Patient B

A 64 year old housewife who is of average weight and has been started on treatment with an oral hypoglycaemic because she has marked urinary frequency and pruritus vulvae.

Prescription: 'Please assess current energy intake and keep it approximately constant, dividing it evenly between 3 main meals with 3 snacks. Not too bright and does not need an exchange portion system anyway. Encourage as much fibre as seems reasonable with 50% or more of energy from carbohydrate. On chlorpropamide 100 mg in the morning. N.B. husband has coeliac disease.'

How often should the patient see the dietitian?

It is usually helpful if a second visit is arranged about four to six weeks after the first. If the patient has questions these can then be answered and if the response to treatment has been poor then the dietitian can look for errors or misunderstandings. Thereafter the frequency of visits will usually be determined by clinical circumstance. If the patient was initially treated with a low calorie diet he will need a further visit for instruction in a maintenance diet when he reaches his target weight. Some diabetologists believe that a dietary review should be undertaken every year or every other year, but if glycaemic and lipaemic control are satisfactory this seems wasteful of both the patient's and the dietitian's time. Obvious exceptions are growing children and pregnant women for whom regular review is mandatory.

Sugar (sucrose), sugar substitutes and special diabetic foods

'Thou shalt not eat sugar' has been one of the dogmas of diabetic management, but is this injunction really necessary? Other simple sugars, for example those in fruit, carry no such embargo. Current evidence suggests that sucrose may be eaten in small amounts, e.g. up to 30 grams daily, provided that it is eaten as part of a high carbohydrate, low fat diet and provided that the sugar is substituted for an isocaloric quantity of other carbohydrate foods such as potato or bread. Allowing small amounts of sugar in this context may enhance the palatability of, and improve compliance with, a high fibre diet. If sucrose is allowed then fructose, which is currently permitted in amounts up to 30 grams daily, should be avoided. Sucrose is 'energy dense' and should still be avoided by those on low calorie diets, and by those who continue to eat a low carbohydrate, low fibre diabetic diet.

Sugar substitutes such as saccharine, acesulfame-K or aspartame can be used by all diabetic patients. Powdered sweeteners are useful for baking or preserves, but contain fructose or sorbitol or sucrose. They should therefore be avoided by those on low calorie diets but others may use them, subject to the limit of 30 grams daily of sucrose or fructose or sorbitol, in conjunction with a high fibre diet.

Special diabetic foods are expensive and often contain fructose or sorbitol as the sweetener. Most of them are unnecessary and best avoided. Products which are suitable and which add some variety to the diet include:

- Carbohydrate-free drinks such as Roses diabetic cordials, Energen One-Cal drinks, Diet-Pepsi and Schweppes Slimline drinks.
- Unsweetened tinned fruits, jams and marmalades. Because they do not contain sugar they do not keep well once opened. These products contain fewer calories than their sweetened equivalents but the carbohydrate and calorie content must still be counted in the patient's daily allowance.
- Sugar-free chewing gum and sweets.

Advice about alcohol and diabetes is given in Chapter 12.

Very low calorie diets (VLCD) and diabetes

Many patients are tempted by manufacturers' claims for the benefits of very low calorie diets (VLCDs) which provide less than 600 calories per day. Unlike the liquid protein VLCD which was marketed in the USA during the 1970s, the modern versions have not been associated with any excess mortality. However, their long-term safety and efficacy are unknown. A VLCD results in greater loss of lean body mass (muscle and bone) than does a conventional reducing diet of 1000 calories and might lead to subsequent osteoporosis. Studies which have compared weight loss in a group of patients on a VLCD with that in a group on a conventional diet suggest that, although weight loss is greater while on a VLCD, subsequent weight gain is also greater so that after one or two years there is no difference in body weight between the two groups.

It is our practice to discourage the use of VLCDs until more is known about their long-term safety. However, diabetic patients, especially those on insulin or oral hypoglycaemics, who insist on using these products, should be offered medical supervision because considerable changes in the dosage of insulin or drug therapy may be needed. Some manufacturers of VLCDs ask patients with diabetes to obtain their doctors' written agreement before supplying the diet. However doctors should be careful about signing such statements unless they are satisfied about the full implications of the diet and are prepared to accept clinical and legal responsibility for the implications of any document which they are asked to sign. In our opinion it is unwise to sign such documents.

Conditions other than diabetes may also be absolute or relative contra-indications to the use of a VLCD. These include patients with cardiac disease, treatment with diuretic or lithium, gout, porphyria, schizophrenia and disorders such as anorexia, bulimia, alcoholism and drug abuse. VLCDs should not be given to children, pregnant women, breast feeding mothers or the elderly.

Diet during intercurrent illness

Any doctor who is called to see an anorexic, nauseated patient must be able to advise on suitable foods or drinks in these circumstances. Unless the patient is vomiting he will usually be able to swallow small quantities of sweet liquids, yoghurts or ice-cream every half-hour. In this way sufficient carbohydrate and calories can be ingested to compensate for the normal diet. Examples of such foods are shown in Appendix 2. Advice on dosage for oral hypoglycaemics and insulin during intercurrent illness is given on pp. 126–127.

Diet and exercise

Exercise will lower the blood glucose concentration because of the energy demands of exercise itself and, in insulin-treated patients, because the vasodilation caused by exercise may result in more rapid absorption of subcutaneously injected insulin. Diabetic patients should be encouraged to take regular exercise but need to know that (a) exercise requires more energy (food), and (b) the effect of exercise on the blood glucose concentration may persist for some hours after exercise has finished. The amount of extra food required will be determined by the nature of the exercise. For example, short-term vigorous exercise like a game of squash will require rapidly absorbed carbohydrate whereas less vigorous but more sustained activity such as a long hill walk will need ingestion of more slowly absorbed, high fibre carbohydrate. There is also considerable individual variation and each patient will have to experiment to find his own requirements. Finger prick blood tests before and after exercise are helpful in some cases.

As a rough and ready rule of thumb:

For short term exercise
- 1 Milky Way or $\frac{1}{2}$ a Mars bar, or
- 4 squares of chocolate, or
- 2 jelly cubes, or
- 200 ml ($\frac{1}{3}$ pint) of pure fruit juice, or
- 200 ml ($\frac{1}{3}$ pint) Coca Cola (**not** diet coke)

If necessary, this can be repeated at half-time, e.g. during a vigorous game of football.

For prolonged exercise
- 2 plain digestive biscuits, or
- 2 Harvest Crunch Bars, or
- 1 Jordans Crunchy Bar, or
- 1 large slice of wholemeal bread, or
- 1 apple and 1 banana, or
- 2 small packs (total 80 gram) of nuts and raisins

Some patients prefer to reduce their insulin dosage instead of, or as well as, eating more. This can work well if exercise is taken at a time appropriate to the action of the insulin which has been reduced. Trial and error will determine what is best for the individual.

■ The patient who will not follow a diet

Most of these patients are overweight and have no intention of changing their lifestyle, but before you give them up as a lost cause there are a few possibilities which are worth considering.

1. **Is the patient illiterate?** Written literature is obviously inappropriate and the patient will need more emphasis on verbal instruction. This can also apply to some patients from **ethnic minority** groups who speak little or no English, and for whom dietary advice must also be tailored to their culture. The BDA produce a leaflet *Food and Diabetes* which is available in Bengali, Gujerati, Urdu and Punjabi.
2. **Was the patient too bemused** to understand? Newly-diagnosed patients may be so taken aback by the diagnosis and its implications that they cannot cope with all the information which is thrown at them. Every patient should have the opportunity of a second visit to the dietitian. Some patients, particularly some of the elderly, learn better in their own homes and a domiciliary visit by the dietitian may well be worth the time and effort involved.
3. **Does whoever cooks the food understand** the diet? There is little to be gained by trying to teach a male patient who doesn't know a saucepan from a food mixer; his wife must be seen as well. Cooks in institutions such as old people's homes and schools may need to be seen.
4. **Do other family members understand** the importance of the diet?

There is evidence that, in some families, it is the husband or father who determines both the type of food and the timing of meals, and the wife's role is to provide what he expects when he expects it. The diet may have to be explained to all members of the family, and some compromises may be needed by all those involved.

5. **Referral to the hospital clinic** may sometimes convince the patient of the importance of diet, and helps to emphasise that the general practitioner is concerned about the situation.

■ What to do if a dietitian is not available

If expert dietary advice is not available to you and your patients there are only two things you can do. The first is to get together with other doctors in a similar position and create a fuss. Write to your Health Authority explaining that a dietetic service is essential for the proper management of diabetes (and other conditions). Enlist the help of local branches of the British Diabetic Association and other patient groups such as the Coeliac Society. Individual patients can write to the Community Health Council and, if necessary, to their Member of Parliament.

While waiting for these efforts to bear fruit, the second thing you will need to do is learn much more about diet and diabetes than you will find in this book. Study the dietetic sections of the books listed at the end of this chapter.

■ Further reading

These books have been written for patients but contain much useful information for those doctors who do not have access to a dietitian.

BDA. *Countdown* (2nd edn). British Diabetic Association, London, 1985. A colour-coded guide to the calorie and carbohydrate content of manufactured foods.

Day J.L. *The Diabetes Handbook*. Thorsons Publishing Group in collaboration with the British Diabetic Association, London, 1986. (There are separate handbooks for non-insulin dependent and insulin dependent patients.)

Diabetes and Nutrition Study Group of the European Association for the Study of Diabetes (1988). Nutritional recommendations for individuals with diabetes mellitus. *Diabetes, Nutrition and Metabolism* **1**, 145–149.

Mann J. *The Diabetics' Diet Book*. Martin Dunitz, London, 1982. Primarily a recipe book with emphasis on a high fibre diet, but with an excellent introductory chapter on dietary principles.

5 ORAL HYPOGLYCAEMIC DRUGS AND INSULIN

Whereas all patients with Type I diabetes require treatment with insulin, some Type II patients can be managed by diet alone and need neither an oral hypoglycaemic agent (OHG) nor insulin. Newly-diagnosed Type II patients should be given an adequate trial in the first instance and the temptation to prescribe an OHG should be resisted. If the diabetes can be controlled by diet alone it helps to emphasise the importance of the diet to the patient. Table 1 shows acceptable blood glucose concentrations tested after fasting and two hours post-prandially. If blood glucose values remain elevated after 4–8 weeks of dietary therapy then treatment with an OHG is indicated. Earlier treatment with an OHG may be indicated in the occasional patient whose troublesome symptoms such as severe pruritis vulvae or considerable urinary frequency are unresponsive to diet alone.

■ Oral hypoglycaemic agents

Approximately one-third of all diabetic patients in this country are on

TABLE 1 TARGET GLUCOSE CONCENTRATIONS FOR TYPE II DIABETES

Test time	Blood glucose concentration (mmol/l)
After fasting	< 7
Two-hour post-prandial	< 11

Note: These criteria may be relaxed for more elderly patients.

OHGs. Two classes of drug are currently available, the **sulphonylureas** and the **biguanides**: they have different modes of action and may therefore be used in combination if indicated. A sulphonylurea should be used in the first instance in those patients who are not grossly overweight, whereas Metformin (the only biguanide available in the UK), which has an anorectic action, is usually preferable in the obese patient.

Oral hypoglycaemics should **not** be used in the following circumstances:

- **Suspected Type I diabetes**
  Although this usually presents in younger patients, it may occur at any age. The onset of symptoms is usually more acute and ketonuria may be present.
- **Pregnancy**
  OHGs should never be used in pregnant patients. The failure of diet indicates the need for insulin.
- **Side effects**
  If there is a past history of unwanted effects or suspected side effects (*vide infra*).

Sulphonylureas

There are many drugs of this class available today and some of the more commonly used ones are listed in Table 2. As they all have the same mode of action, they should not be used in combination. Sulphonylureas stimulate the release of insulin by the pancreatic beta cells, and also have a number of extra-pancreatic effects, such as increasing insulin-mediated uptake of glucose in peripheral tissues. As pancreatic islet cell function is needed for sulphonylurea action, **there is no place for the use of these drugs in Type I diabetes.**

Indications and contraindications

The main indication for an OHG is in the patient who fails to respond to an adequate trial of dietary therapy. The need to continue the prescribed diet must be emphasised — all too often patients believe that the tablet enables them to return to their old eating habits. Treatment should be started with a low dose and the dose increased according to the response. The aims of treatment are to abolish symptoms, achieve satisfactory glycaemic control and to avoid side effects of the drug. Acceptable fasting and

TABLE 2 COMMONLY USED ORAL HYPOGLYCAEMIC AGENTS

Proper name	Trade name	Tablet size (mg)	Duration of action (hrs)	Starting dose (mg)	Maximum dose (mg)
Sulphonylureas					
Chlorpropamide†	Diabinese, Melitase	{100, 250}	Up to 60	100	500
Glibenclamide†	Daonil, Semi-Daonil, Euglucon	2.5, 5.0	5–20 +	2.5	20 (divided)
Gliclazide	Diamicron	80	5–16	40	320 (divided)
Glipizide	Glibenese, Minodiab	5.0	5–12	2.5	20 (divided)
Tolbutamide	Pramidex, Rastinon	500	5–12	500	3000 (divided)
Biguanides					
Metformin★	Glucophage, Orabet	{500, 850}	12–24	500	1700 (divided)

† Care required in older patients and those with renal impairment.
★ Do not use if renal or hepatic impairment or in hypoxic patients.

two-hour post-prandial blood glucose results are given in Table 1. It is advisable to wait for at least 7–10 days before increasing the dose.

Which sulphonylurea?

The selection of a sulphonylurea is often a matter of personal preference, but in making the decision the following points should be considered.

1. *Pharmacological properties*
   The major biochemical abnormality in most patients with Type II diabetes is resistance to the action of insulin, and consequently the blood glucose concentration is higher than normal at all times of the day and night. In theory, therefore, it would be logical to use a drug with a duration of action of at least 24 hours. However, long-acting drugs such as chlorpropamide may accumulate in the body and caution is required when they are prescribed for those with impaired renal function, and some doctors advise that chlorpropamide should not be used in the elderly.

2. *Potency*
   There have been several reports of serious hypoglycaemic events in patients treated with Glibenclamide, which is probably the most potent member of this group of drugs. It may be best reserved for those patients whose control has been inadequate on full doses of less potent sulphonylureas. Daily doses in excess of 5 mg are best given in divided doses to minimise the risk of hypoglycaemia.

3. *Cost*
   OHGs vary greatly in price — see current issues of MIMS or BNF.

4. *Weight gain*
   Patients experiencing difficulty with weight loss may be less prone to gain weight on Gliclazide than on other sulphonylureas.

5. *Other medical conditions*
   Patients with renal impairment should be prescribed a drug with a short duration of action such as Tolbutamide, or a drug which is metabolised in the liver, such as Gliclazide. However, those drugs which are metabolised in the liver must be used with caution in patients with hepatic disease, but are not contraindicated if liver function is stable and blood glucose concentrations are monitored regularly.

Side effects

The commonest unwanted effect of this group of drugs is hypoglycaemia which may be prolonged and relapsing, especially in older patients (see

Chapter 14). Other side effects are rare, but include allergic skin reactions and gastrointestinal problems such as nausea, vomiting and diarrhoea, blood dyscrasias and hepatic damage. Such effects may be dose related, so there is no indication to exceed the maximum doses given in Table 2 because this increases the likelihood of side effects without improving efficacy.

One recognised side effect with Chlorpropamide (and occasionally Tolbutamide) is facial flushing after ingestion of alcohol. Although not serious, this can be distressing and embarrassing for the patient and an alternative sulphonylurea may be prescribed.

Chlorpropamide can cause hyponatraemia, especially if used in conjunction with combined Amiloride/Thiazide preparations. The serum sodium should be checked at the annual review.

Drug interactions

Interactions between sulphonylureas and other commonly used medications may occur and it is important to be aware of this possibility. The main interactions are listed in Table 3. Should it be necessary to prescribe or withdraw any of these drugs, then the patient should be advised to monitor either urine or blood tests more frequently.

Primary and secondary drug failures

Primary failures (i.e. patients who *never* show a therapeutic response after 4–8 weeks of drug therapy) may occasionally occur in patients who are actually Type I but who present as if they have Type II diabetes. Other causes include a failure to continue on the prescribed diet when the OHG

TABLE 3 DRUG INTERACTIONS AND SULPHONYLUREAS

1. Drugs which may **increase** hypoglycaemic action:

Salicylates	Propranolol
Phenylbutazone	Alcohol
Sulphonamides	Clofibrate, Bezafibrate
Oral anticoagulants	Monoamine oxidase inhibitors

2. Drugs which may **reduce** hypoglycaemic action:

Glucocorticoids	Frusemide, Bumetanide
Oestrogens	Rifampicin
Thiazides	

is prescribed, or a more severe form of Type II diabetes. Secondary failures (i.e. worsening glycaemic control after a satisfactory initial response) may indicate a progressive loss of islet cell mass and therefore a reduced response to the drug. Whatever the cause of the drug failure, a change in therapy is usually indicated. The addition of Metformin may restore glycaemic control in patients with secondary failure, especially in overweight patients. The problem of inadequate control in patients on full doses of a sulphonylurea and Metformin is considered in Chapter 15.

Temporary drug failure may occur during stressful situations such as an acute illness; in such cases insulin may be required until there is a return to basal conditions, when OHG therapy may be resumed.

█ Biguanides

Metformin is the only biguanide which is avaiable in the UK. Although some islet cell function appears to be necessary for its action, it does not stimulate insulin release and does not cause hypoglycaemia. As with the sulphonylureas, Metformin should not be used in patients with Type I diabetes.

Indications and contraindications

The role of biguanides has been questioned in recent years because their use has been associated with **lactic acidosis** and it was for this reason Phenformin was withdrawn. However, there is undoubtedly a role for Metformin in the management of the obese Type II diabetic patient who remains hyperglycaemic despite treatment with diet, or diet and sulphonylurea. Renal impairment is the main risk factor for the development of lactic acidosis in patients treated with **Metformin** which **should not be used in those whose serum creatinine concentration is above the upper limit of the normal range**. It should also be avoided in patients who have other risk factors for lactic acidosis, i.e. hepatic disease or cardiorespiratory disease severe enough to cause hypoxia.

Other side effects
The commonest are those affecting gastrointestinal tract and include:

- a metallic taste in the mouth
- anorexia (which can be beneficial in the obese patient!)
- flatulence, nausea and occasionally vomiting
- diarrhoea

Problems with flatulence and nausea can often be avoided or minimised by giving the drug after food and by building up the dose gradually. These measures do not usually help the diarrhoea which may respond to small doses of Codeine but which often necessitates withdrawal of the drug.

■ Other hypoglycaemic medications

A number of naturally occurring fibres and herbal remedies have been studied in patients with Type II diabetes. Of these, the best known is guar gum, a viscous fibre which reduces the post-prandial peak of glucose absorption by delaying gastric emptying and possibly by interfering with the process of digestion. Guar is prescribable, and can be sprinkled on food. However, it may cause gastrointestinal side effects, such as flatulence and diarrhoea, and clinical trials have not shown conclusively that it is of major benefit.

■ Insulins

The large number of insulins currently available can cause confusion amongst prescribers, and it is useful to start with some general statements:

- Try to be familiar with a small number of preparations. Insulins used in your local diabetic clinic would be a logical start.
- Think of insulin action as being of **short** (e.g. soluble type of insulin), **intermediate** (e.g. Isophane) or **long** (e.g. Ultralente) duration of action.
- There is a trend towards increasing usage of human insulin. However, at least one manufacturer has stated that purified beef insulins will continue to be available: these are listed in Table 4.

Pharmacology of insulin

Currently available insulins are of bovine, porcine or 'human' origin. Bovine and porcine insulins differ from human insulin in only three or one amino acids, respectively, in the alpha chain. True insulin allergy is extremely rare and, despite the many published papers on insulin antibodies, these are only occasionally of clinical importance. Thus, to the patient there is usually little difference between human, bovine or porcine insulins. Human insulin can either be manufactured biosynthetically by recombinant DNA technology (Lilly insulins), or semi-synthetically by enzyme modification of porcine insulin (Nordisk and Novo insulins). It is likely that the use of human insulins will continue to grow in the next decade.

Insulin action *(Tables 4 and 5)*

The duration of action of subcutaneously injected insulins may be described under the following headings.

Short
Soluble insulins were the first to be available in 1922, and are still commonly used today: these are the only insulins that may be given intramuscularly and intravenously as well as subcutaneously. When injected s.c., onset of action is within an hour, peak action 2–4 hours and duration up to 8 hours after injections. Short acting insulins are most commonly used in combination with an intermediate acting insulin in Type I diabetic patients.

Intermediate
The addition of protamine (e.g. in Isophane insulin) or Zinc (e.g. in Lente type insulins) delays the absorption and prolongs the duration of action of

TABLE 4 HIGHLY PURIFIED BEEF INSULINS

Insulin*	Approximate action (hours)		
	Onset	Maximum action	Duration
Short acting			
Hypurin Neutral	$\frac{1}{2}$	2–4	7
Intermediate acting			
Hypurin Isophane	2	6–10	22
Long acting			
Hypurin Lente	2	8–12	26–30
Hypurin PZI	5	10–18	32

Note: onset, maximum action and duration are approximate and vary between individuals and injection sites used. Neutral should not be mixed with PZI in the same syringe.

*All manufactured by C.P. Pharmaceuticals.

TABLE 5 HIGHLY PURIFIED PORCINE AND HUMAN INSULINS

Insulin	Manufacturer	Onset	Approximate action (hours)	
			Maximum	Duration
Short acting				
Human Actrapid	Novo	$\frac{1}{2}$	2–4	8
Humulin S	Lilly	$\frac{1}{2}$	1–3	7
Velosulin	Nordisk	$\frac{1}{2}$	1–3	8
Intermediate acting				
Human Protophane	Novo	2	4–10	22
Humulin I	Lilly	1	3–8	18
Human Monotard	Novo	3	8–14	22
Insulatard	Nordisk	2	4–12	22
Long acting				
Humulin ZN	Lilly	3	6–14	24
Human Ultratard	Novo	4	8–20	28–30

Note: All the above are available as Human insulins. Nordisk insulins are also available as highly purified porcine.

subcutaneously injected insulin. Intermediate acting insulins (see Tables 4 and 5) may be used once or twice daily depending on the regimen chosen.

Long

These insulins (e.g. Ultralente and Protamine Zinc insulin) have a duration of action of 24 hours or more and are used once daily, usually in combination with a short acting insulin given before one or more of the main meals.

Pre-mixed insulins

A number of pre-mixed insulins are now available (Table 6) and are usually given twice daily, before breakfast and before the main evening meal. The use of these mixed insulins is increasing, especially in older patients who have difficulty in mixing two insulins in one syringe. The action of these insulins depends on the proportion of soluble and Isophane in the mixture. Thus Initard (50:50 soluble/isophane) will have approximately equal action in the morning and afternoon when given before breakfast, whereas Humulin M1 (10:90 soluble/isophane) will have a greater action in the afternoon.

Essentials of insulin administration

Strength

All insulin in the UK is now U100; therefore 1 ml contains 100 units, and the standard 10 ml vial contains 1000 units.

Syringes

Two sizes of syringe are generally available in glass or plastic: these are the 0.5 ml (50 unit) and 1 ml (100 units) syringes. The 50 unit syringe has 50 divisions with one division on the syringe equalling one unit. (The word 'mark' is best avoided as it can give rise to confusion with many patients, being reminiscent of the U40 and U80 days when marks and units were always different.) However, the 100 unit syringe also has 50 divisions with one division of the syringe equalling 2 units.

Both plastic and glass syringe are prescribable, and evidence suggests that the plastic syringes can safely be reused by the same patient until the needle becomes blunt or the markings indistinct. If they are reused the cap should be replaced on the needle, and they should be stored in a dry, cool, clean place. Any risk of infection from reusing syringes appears to be minimal. Glass syringes should be stored in industrial methylated spirit between usage. For the visually handicapped, the pre-set or click-count

TABLE 6 PRE-MIXED INSULINS

Name	Manufacturer	Short acting component	Intermediate acting component	Ratio short: intermediate
Initard	Nordisk	Velosulin	Insulatard	50:50
Mixtard	Nordisk	Velosulin	Insulatard	30:70
Actraphane	Novo	Actrapid	Protophane	30:70
Humulin M1	Lilly	Humulin S	Humulin I	10:90
Humulin M2		Humulin S	Humulin I	20:80
Humulin M3		Humulin S	Humulin I	30:70
Humulin M4		Humulin S	Humulin I	40:60

Note: All are available as human insulins. Nordisk insulins are also available as highly purified porcine.

glass syringes are available. There are also magnifying glasses which clip onto plastic syringes.

Sites
Three main sites are recommended: the **upper thighs and buttocks**, the **upper arm** and **abdomen**. Rotation between sites is advisable, though it should be remembered that absorption rates may vary slightly at different sites, being fastest from the abdomen.

Drawing up insulin
Detailed descriptions are available in the educational literature supplied by manufacturers and the BDA — see Appendix 5. In summary, **it is important to inject the equivalent number of units of air into the insulin bottle before drawing up the insulin**.
   If clear and cloudy insulins are being mixed:

1. inject the correct number of units of air into air space of the cloudy insulin bottle
2. inject the correct units of air into the clear insulin bottle
3. draw up the clear insulin and expel any air bubbles
4. draw up the correct dose of cloudy insulin

Technique
There is no need to use an alcohol swab to cleanse the skin, as long as the area is clean. A brisk insertion of the needle at 90° to the skin is the least painful method.

Starting insulin

The most important aim of insulin therapy must be the improvement of the patient's sense of well-being by removing symptoms of hyperglycaemia whilst avoiding the most unpleasant acute side effect — that of symptomatic hypoglycaemia. An important secondary aim is the achievement and maintenance of good glycaemic control in the hope of reducing the chances of developing long-term complications. The desirable or acceptable standard of glycaemic control may therefore vary according to the age of the patient: we would not aim for as strict control in a 75 year old patient who had failed on oral agents as in a 15 year old with newly-diagnosed Type I diabetes.
   Three cases are now presented to demonstrate the uses of different insulin regimens.

Case 1

A 24 year old man with a three-week history of thirst, polyuria and a 5 kg weight loss. Urinalysis 2% glycosuria, trace of ketones. Fasting blood glucose 17.8 mmol/l. **Diagnosis**: Type I diabetes. At the hospital clinic he is seen by the dietitian, instructed in home blood glucose monitoring and started on Insulatard 12 units in the morning and 8 units in the evening (Insulatard is an isophane, intermediate acting insulin). Over the next few months his diabetes remains relatively stable and he is seen at home by the diabetes specialist nurse. Follow-up is then arranged at the local mini-clinic with annual reviews at the hospital.

Mini-clinic visit 1: when first seen at the mini-clinic, home blood glucose monitoring results (average) were as listed in Table 7. As can be seen, these are all elevated and it was, therefore, decided to increase each insulin dosage. **Advice**: Insulatard increased to 14 units in the morning, 10 units in the evening.

Mini-clinic visit 2: the results of home blood glucose monitoring are shown in Table 7 for the second visit. Although there has been some improvement, especially before tea, the blood glucose readings at other times remained unacceptably high. **Advice**: from this profile it appears that the patient needs a short acting insulin mixed with the Insulatard, which is an intermediate acting insulin. If his dose of Insulatard was simply increased, it is quite probable that he may become hypoglycaemic before tea. A small dose of Velosulin, a short acting insulin, was therefore added to the intermediate acting insulin, as shown in Table 7.

Mini-clinic visit 3: as shown in the table, results of home blood glucose monitoring were much improved. However, the blood glucose before lunch remains high and the patient is advised that the aim of the insulin treatment is to achieve results of 4–8 mmol/l at all times. **Advice**: the morning dosage of Velosulin is increased further to achieve a lower pre-lunch blood glucose.

TABLE 7 INSULIN ADJUSTMENTS FOR CASE 1

Visit	Insulin dosage (units) a.m.	p.m.	Fasting	Before lunch	Before tea	Before bed	Advice a.m.	p.m.
1	I 12	I 8	15	17	11	17	I 14	I 10
2	I 14	I 10	11	17	7	11	V 4 / I 14	V 4 / I 10
3	V 4 / I 14	V 4 / I 10	9	11	4.5	7	V 6 / I 14	V 4 / I 10
4	V 6 / I 14	V 4 / I 10	6	4.5	7	7	Continuing same dose	

Home blood glucose monitoring (mmol/l)

Key: V = Velosulin; I = Insulatard.

Mini-clinic visit 4: most results are in the target range and the advice is therefore to continue on the present dosage with regular home blood glucose monitoring.

Comment: appropriate adjustments in short and intermediate acting insulins lead to satisfactory control in this case.

Case 2

A 55 year old woman with Type II diabetes, within 10% of ideal body weight. Fasting blood glucose 12.8 mmol/l, HbA_1C 12.5% (non-diabetic range: 6–8%), remains symptomatic on maximum doses of OHGs. She agrees to change to insulin, but in view of her anxiety about injections and the possibility of needing to mix insulins, it is decided to start her on a pre-mixed insulin. **Plan**: she initially sees the dietitian for review as alterations may be needed in the patient changing from OHGs to insulin (see Chapter 4). It is decided to start her on a pre-mixed insulin, for example, Humulin M1 12 units in the morning, 8 units in the evening. She also receives instruction in home blood glucose monitoring.

Visit 1: one week later she attends for review and the results of HBGM for this and subsequent visits are shown in Table 8. As all results are above the target range at this visit and she has experienced no episodes suggestive of hypoglycaemia, the advice is to increase her dosage of insulin to 14 units in the morning, 10 units in the evening.

Visit 2: at this visit, one week following Visit 1, she complains that she has been feeling rather hungry when she wakes up. However, as can be seen from the table, the results before lunch and before bed remain a little high. An increase in the dose of Humulin M1 at this stage might lead to hypoglycaemia before tea and fasting. It was, therefore, decided to change her to Humulin M3 which has a higher proportion of shorter acting insulin and she was left on the same dosage.

TABLE 8 INSULIN ADJUSTMENTS FOR CASE 2

Visit	Insulin dosage (units)		Home blood glucose monitoring (mmol/l)				Advice	
	a.m.	p.m.	Fasting	Before lunch	Before tea	Before bed	a.m.	p.m.
1	M1 12	M1 8	7	11	9	17	M1 14	M1 10
2	M1 14	M1 10	4.5	11	7	11	M3 14	M3 10
3	M3 14	M3 10	7	9	9	9	M3 16	M3 12
4	M3 16	M3 12	6	7	7	6	Continuing same dose	

Key: M1 = Humulin M1; M3 = Humulin M3.

Visit 3: the effect of the last change in insulin can be seen in that pre-lunch and before bed blood glucose results are improved, though all the results are now a little above the target range. The advice is, therefore, to increase both morning and evening Humulin M3 by 2 units.

Visit 4: the patient feels well and all results are in the target range.

Comment: pre-mixed insulins can be very useful in certain cases though, as in this case, a change in the prescription may be necessary to achieve optimum glood glucose control. Target ranges for blood glucose should be as for a patient with Type I diabetes in someone of this age group.

Case 3

A seventy-five year old woman with Type II diabetes, 20% overweight, fasting blood glucose 15.2 mmol/l; HbA$_1$C 14% who remains symptomatic despite maximum doses of oral agents. Twice before she has refused to consider insulin therapy, but on this occasion agreed to try therapy for a short period of time as she is feeling so thirsty and lethargic. This is a common problem and the patient may be helped with one injection of long acting insulin daily. You arrange for the district nurse to visit her at home and she is started on Ul-tratard 14 units daily. The patient continues to perform urine testing and the district nurse checks the fasting blood glucose when she arrives to supervise insulin injections. The dosage is gradually increased according to fasting blood glucose results and within a few weeks the patient is giving her own injections and feeling considerably better. At a dose of 26 units daily she has fasting blood glucose results around 7 mmol/l and has no symptoms of hyperglycaemia. It is also important to re-emphasise the need to adhere to the diet if further weight gain is not to occur.

Points to note for starting insulin therapy
1. Newly-diagnosed diabetic patients should be encouraged to give their own injections from the first day of therapy.
2. There is no magic formula to calculate the correct dosage of insulin. A trial and error approach is used but it is best to start with a low dose to avoid frightening hypoglycaemia in the early days of insulin therapy.
3. Newly-diagnosed Type I diabetic patients may go through the 'honeymoon period' with reducing insulin requirements during the first few months of treatment.
4. In Type II diabetes, when a basal insulin supplement is used (e.g. Ultralente), the injection may be given at any time of the day, and if control is unsatisfactory, soluble insulin may be added before one or more meals, if required.

Special devices

Pen injection devices
A number of pen injection devices are now available. The most commonly used is the 'Novo Pen' into which is fitted a cartridge of insulin. The Novopen 1 will take cartridges of Human Actrapid, whereas the Novopen 2 will also take Human Actraphane and Protophane. This kind of regimen is popular with many patients who find the injections less painful and, in addition, report that the use of this device leads to increased flexibility of lifestyle. The usual regimen with the Novopen 1 is to take the short acting insulin via the pen before each of the three main meals and then to give a longer acting insulin at night. This latter insulin may be an Isophane type (e.g. Protophane) or an ultra long acting insulin such as Ultratard.

Continuous subcutaneous insulin infusion (CSII)
At present the use of CSII is not increasing because of the many problems that have been associated with this mode of insulin delivery. It is unlikely that supervision of such treatment will ever be the task of a mini-clinic. The technique uses a continuous basal infusion of insulin given by a syringe pump which can be boosted at meal times by the patient. Such regimens require intensive home blood glucose monitoring and a high degree of compliance by the patient.

■ Further reading

Oral hypoglycaemic agents

Chan A.W. and MacFarlane I.A. (1988). The pharmacology of oral agents used to treat diabetes mellitus. *Practical Diabetes* 5, 59–64.

MacFarlane I.A. (1988). The treatment of non-insulin dependent diabetes (Editorial). *Practical Diabetes* **5**, 52.

Insulin

Holman R.R., Steemson J. and Turner R.C. (1987). Sulphonylurea failure in Type II diabetes: treatment with a basal insulin supplement. *Diabetic Medicine* **4**, 457–462.

6 'GOOD DIABETIC CONTROL'

■ What is 'good diabetic control'?

We all talk about 'diabetic control', but what do we mean when we say that a patient's diabetes is 'well controlled' or 'badly controlled'?

The ideal would be to have achieved a state of normal metabolic homeostasis with normal concentrations of glucose, lipids, insulin and other regulatory hormones without having caused any side effects. In practice this ideal state is probably only attainable in some diet-treated, obese patients who reduce their weight to the ideal level for their height and age. In the great majority of cases some **compromise will be necessary**.

What we accept as a satisfactory standard of diabetic control may be influenced by many factors; examples of these are outlined below.

Age

In an 80 year old our main priorities will be to alleviate symptoms without causing side effects, and we will be less concerned about the value of good control in preventing long-term complications.

Occupation

The irregular, and frequently unpredictable, working hours and physical exercise in jobs such as farming may make it impossible to achieve the same degree of control as in someone with a more regular daily routine.

Personality and motivation

However hard we may try to motivate our patients we have to accept that there are some who will never put in the time and effort required to achieve good diabetic control. The patient's educational and social background may influence his attitude to his diabetes, as may the support, or lack of support, from parents and other family members.

The diabetes itself

Some patients have 'difficult diabetes'. It is not always the patient who is difficult!

Other medical conditions

Blood glucose concentrations can be greatly influenced by intercurrent illness, both physical and mental, and at these times we may have to accept less than optimal diabetic control. Pregnancy is an indication for excellent diabetic control (Chapter 11).

From these examples the reader will understand that there is no simple definition of good diabetic control. What is acceptable in one patient may not be so in another, and what is acceptable in any given patient may alter from time to time as a result of other medical or social circumstances.

> We can define *good diabetic control* as being:
> As near normal metabolic homeostasis as can be achieved without significant side effects at any given time.

■ The assessment of diabetic control

There is no single measure of diabetic control and the doctor must take account of all the available evidence which comprises symptoms of hyper- or hypoglycaemia, change in body weight, the results of home monitoring by the patient of urine or blood glucose concentrations, and the results of laboratory investigations (Table 1). All of this evidence must be considered; for example a normal glycosylated haemoglobin result does not indicate good control if the patient is having frequent attacks of hypoglycaemia. The assessment of diabetic control implies more than just glycaemic homeo-stasis, and account must also be taken of measurements of lipid metabolism (see Chapter 13).

Home blood glucose monitoring by the patient

Home blood glucose monitoring (HBGM) has been a major advance in the management of many insulin treated patients. There is probably little to

TABLE 1 METHODS OF ASSESSING DIABETIC CONTROL

Symptoms
- hypoglycaemia
- hyperglycaemia
  e.g. thirst, polyuria, weight loss, boils, pruritus vulvae, cramp

Home monitoring
- results of blood or urine tests

Surgery tests
- fasting blood glucose
- two-hour post-prandial blood glucose
- ketonuria if hyperglycaemia
- measures of longer term glycaemic control, e.g. glycosylated haemoglobin
- serum lipid concentrations

Always consider ALL the available evidence

choose between the different makes of reagent strip, but they are all expensive and the availability of a strip which can be cut in half, such as the BM 1-44 strip, may be regarded as an advantage. Most of the strips can be read by eye and a meter is only necessary for patients with defective colour vision or severely impaired visual acuity.

The results obtained with HBGM strips depend on the care with which the strip is used. They should not be prescribed until the patient has been instructed in their correct usage, and it is the responsibility of the prescriber to ensure that training is provided. The patient should then demonstrate his ability to perform the technique and obtain a correct reading. If this is not done, dangerously misleading results may be obtained. The results obtained with reagent strips are not as consistently reliable as the measurement of blood glucose concentrations in a laboratory. **The diagnosis of diabetes should not be based on the result of a strip designed for HBGM** — a simultaneous sample should be sent to the laboratory for subsequent confirmation of the diagnosis. For the same reason it is unwise to rely solely on a strip result if there may be medico-legal implications, e.g. in the diagnosis of hypoglycaemia following a road traffic accident.

The results of HBGM should be recorded in a book (Figure 1) to make interpretation easier. Record books are usually freely available from the local hospital clinic, and are also provided by a number of pharmaceutical companies (see Appendix 5). If the diabetes is stable then one test each day, at a different time each day, will be sufficient. Some patients prefer to do four tests on each of two days every week, but this may lead to bias if they

Month: APRIL

Date	Insulin Units or Tablets AM	PM	Before B'kfast	Mid morning	Before lunch	Before Supper	Before Bed	Diet Formula and Notes
1	A8 M16	A4 M8	4					
2					7			
3						6		
4							9	
5			7		4			Tennis a.m.
6						4		
7							13	
8			6		5			
9								
10						7		
11							11	
12			7					
13					4			
14						9		
15							11	PM Actrapid needs increase

Average 6   5   6½   11

Month

Date	Insulin Units or Tablets AM	PM	Before B'kfast	Mid-morning	Before Lunch	Before Supper	Before Bed	Diet Formula and Notes
16	A8 M16	A6 M8	5					
17					7			
18							10	Tummy bug →
19	A10 M18	A8 M10	13		11	11	9	
20	"	"	9				10	
21	A8 M18	A6 M8	7		6	8	5	
22	A8 M16	"	5			4		
23					4	6		
24								
25			6				8	
26								
27					7			
28						5	14	Out to dinner!
29			6					
30						3		Tennis p.m.
31							7	

A = Actrapid   M = Monotard

FIGURE 1 A METHOD FOR RECORDING THE RESULTS OF HOME BLOOD GLUCOSE MONITORING (SEE TEXT FOR DISCUSSION).

choose to do the tests on atypical days, e.g. only on days when they are not at work. The most useful information is obtained from tests done before meals and before bed, at which times the results should be as near normal as possible. It can sometimes be helpful to work out the average result at each time of day before deciding if a change in insulin dose is appropriate — see Figure 1. Additional tests may be done depending on circumstances, e.g. if hypoglycaemia is suspected but the symptoms are not entirely typical, or following exercise. The testing will need to be more often than once a day if insulin requirements are changing rapidly, e.g. during inter-current illness (see Figure 1) or during pregnancy.

It is essential that the clinician should study the record book carefully at each consultation, reviewing all results since the last visit. If this is not done the patient may feel that the results are of little or no significance, and that the value of obtaining and recording the results is not worth the effort.

Reagent strips for HBGM can now be prescribed by general prac-titioners in the United Kingdom. They are much more expensive than urine test strips and DHSS guidelines state that they are primarily intended for insulin treated patients. They are only occasionally required in non-insulin treated patients. Poor diabetic control is not in itself an indication for the prescription of HBGM strips. However, HBGM may be the only way of obtaining the information needed to improve diabetic control in an insulin treated patient, whereas this is rarely true of poorly controlled diabetes in patients who are not on insulin.

Home monitoring of urine glucose and ketones

The measurement of urine glucose concentrations provides an indirect assessment of degree of hyperglycaemia. Glucose only appears in the urine when the blood glucose concentration exceeds about 10 mmol/l, so the absence of glycosuria does not necessarily imply good glycaemic control. The renal threshold increases with age and with decreasing glomerular function. Some patients have an abnormally low renal threshold and will always show glycosuria even if their blood glucose concentrations are in the normal range. The urine glucose concentration is a reflection of what has been happening to blood glucose concentrations since the patient last passed urine, which may have been some hours previously and may include a period of peak hyperglycaemia following a meal. This problem can be minimised by testing a double-voided sample, but this is inconvenient for the patient and may still give spurious results if there is a degree of urinary retention with incomplete voiding, as may occur with prostatic hyper-trophy or autonomic neuropathy.

Despite these limitations, home monitoring of urine glucose concentrations can still provide useful information in most patients with Type II diabetes treated with diet or oral hypoglycaemic drugs. As with HBGM, the following guidelines should be followed.

1. The patient should be instructed in the use of the reagent strips and should demonstrate his ability to use the strips correctly.
2. The results should be recorded in a record book.
3. There is little to choose between the different strips available. The use of the strip employed in the local hospital can avoid confusion if the patient needs referral to the out-patient clinic or admission to hospital. Clinitest tablets are almost obsolete. They are time-consuming to use and, because they measure reducing substances rather than glucose, they may give false positive results (see p. 128).

With urine monitoring, as opposed to HBGM, it is sometimes helpful to test a mid-morning or two-hour postprandial sample because this may be the only time at which the blood glucose concentration exceeds the renal threshold and a positive result at these times suggests that the blood glucose concentration has been above the renal threshold of approximately 10 mmol/l.

Urine tests in insulin treated patients are of much less value than blood tests in that they cannot detect asymptomatic hypoglycaemia and the results may be meaningless if the blood glucose concentration is fluctuating rapidly. However it is reasonable to allow older patients with well controlled, stable diabetes to continue with the urine test that they have been doing for years, particularly if they show any reluctance to learn HBGM. Measurement of urine ketone concentrations is not often needed, but patients with unstable Type I diabetes should be given 'Ketostix' and advised to test for ketones during intercurrent illness or if blood tests reveal significant hyperglycaemia, e.g. greater than about 14 mmol/l.

Urine and blood tests in the surgery or clinic

Urine tests

Testing for glycosuria in the clinic is useful only in so far as a major discrepancy with the patient's own results may indicate that the tests are not being carried out correctly or that the results recorded in the home monitoring record are a complete fabrication! If the urine test is a double-voided sample and timed to coincide with a blood test it may provide useful information about an abnormal renal threshold for glucose.

Testing for protein is essential and should be done routinely at the annual review. Testing for very small quantities of albuminuria ('microalbuminuria' — see Chapter 8) can provide information about the earliest stages of diabetic nephropathy and is also a marker for more generalised vascular disease. This test is likely to be used increasingly in the future. Some laboratories require an early morning urine sample while others prefer a timed overnight collection.

All surgeries and clinics should stock 'Ketostix' to test for ketonuria, even though the test is not routinely required at follow-up visits. **Ketonuria in a poorly controlled patient or in a newly diagnosed patient usually indicates insulin deficiency and requires urgent action** (see Chapter 7).

Blood tests

A single, random measurement of blood glucose concentration in the surgery is of limited value in the management of insulin treated diabetes, except when the result is unexpectedly very high or low. However in non-insulin treated patients the diurnal excursions in blood glucose concentration are very much smaller than in those treated with insulin, and a two-hour post-prandial blood glucose concentration of less than 11 mmol/l usually indicates satisfactory glycaemic control in those treated with diet alone or with a long-acting oral hypoglycaemic (OHG) such as chlorpropamide. Some doctors prefer to measure a fasting blood glucose concentration for patients on OHGs, as this is a good measure of overall glycaemic control, but does entail a small risk of hypoglycaemia while travelling to the surgery.

Most laboratories now provide assays which give a measure of the average level of glycaemia during the preceding weeks. The most widely available test is the glycosylated haemoglobin analysis which is described in the next section. Other such tests include measurement of fructosamine and glycosylated albumin.

Glycosylated haemoglobin

What it is

Glycosylated haemoglobin (GlyHb) is haemoglobin to which glucose molecules have become attached as red cells circulate in the bloodstream in contact with glucose. The amount of glucose which becomes attached to the haemoglobin molecules is proportional to the average prevailing blood glucose concentration. The higher the blood glucose concentration the greater the proportion of haemoglobin which will be glycosylated.

What it tells us

Because the average red blood cell circulates for about 120 days, the amount of GlyHb is a measure of the average blood glucose concentration during the preceding 6–8 weeks.

Some problems in interpreting results

1. The result will be influenced by conditions which affect the life span of red blood cells. For example the GlyHb will fall if the proportion of young red cells is increased, as occurs with haemolysis, during treatment of iron deficiency anaemia or during the second trimester of pregnancy.
2. Depending on the method of assay the presence of abnormal haemoglobins or persistent fetal haemoglobin may give abnormally high results.
3. Some assay methods will give abnormally high results in uraemic patients (due to the presence of carbamylated haemoglobin), in patients treated with high dose aspirin (due to acetylated haemoglobin) and in alcoholics (due to haemoglobin which is linked to acetaldehyde).
4. Some methods will give abnormally high results if there is a delay in processing the sample and the blood was taken at a time when the blood glucose concentration happened to be high. In these circumstances the glucose in the blood sample continues to bind to haemoglobin during transit to the laboratory. The binding which occurs is relatively weak or 'labile' and this labile glucose can be removed by dialysis or saline incubation. However not all laboratories remove the weakly bound glucose, and this may affect the results if samples are sent in by post with an inevitable delay of at least a day before the sample is processed.

When to measure GlyHb

Most assays are time-consuming and therefore expensive. There is no point in measuring it if control is known to have been poor in the last two months, or if there is no intention of trying to improve glycaemic control as in a very elderly asymptomatic patient whose two-hour postprandial blood glucose result is acceptable.

The chief indication is the insulin treated patient whose blood and urine results suggest that control is reasonable. Two or three measurements each year are usually sufficient in these patients. In non-insulin treated patients an annual measurement is usually sufficient if the fasting or two-hour postprandial blood glucose results and home monitoring tests are satisfactory.

Interpreting GlyHb results

The result is usually expressed as a percentage of the total haemoglobin:

$$\frac{\text{GlyHb concentration}}{\text{Total Hb concentration}} \times 100$$

The normal reference range depends on the assay method and varies from one laboratory to another.

GlyHb is not a 'gold standard' of glycaemic control and the results should always be interpreted in the light of all the available evidence. A common problem in clinical practice is the finding of a high GlyHb result when the patient's HBGM results suggest good control. The commonest explanation is that the HBGM results are wrong. Either the patient has used the strips incorrectly or sometimes the recorded results are entirely fictitious. However, it may be that the GlyHb assay has given a spuriously high result due to the presence of an abnormal haemoglobin or one of the other causes discussed above. Conversely a GlyHb result in the normal reference range does not necessarily indicate good glycaemic control because the patient may be oscillating between hyper- and hypoglycaemia. A good GlyHb result in the presence of daytime blood glucose results which are unexpectedly high should alert the clinician to the possibility of asymptomatic nocturnal hypoglycaemia.

■ Summary

The key points for assessing whether a patient's diabetes is well controlled are outlined below.

1. Good diabetic control means more than just good blood test results. It also means the absence of hypoglycaemia and absence of side effects of drugs. It means good glycaemic control and also good lipid homeostasis.
2. What constitutes good or acceptable diabetic control will vary from one patient to another. There is no single gold standard.
3. Patients must be properly instructed in the use of reagent strips for home monitoring of blood or urine glucose concentrations. If this is not done then dangerously misleading results may be obtained. The results are of greatest value if they are recorded in a book designed for this purpose.
4. Glycosylated haemoglobin measurements are an expensive but very valuable measure of average levels of glycaemia during the preceding two months. Spurious values can occur and the results should always be interpreted in the light of all the available evidence.

■ **Further reading**

Ashby J.P., Deacon A.C. and Frier B.M. (1985). Glycosylated haemoglobin: measurement and clinical interpretation. *Diabetic Medicine* **2**, 83–85.

Day J.L. *The Diabetes Handbook (Insulin Dependent Diabetes)*. Thorsons Publishing Group in collaboration with The British Diabetic Association, London, 1986. Gives useful practical advice on home blood and urine glucose monitoring.

7 HYPOGLYCAEMIA AND HYPERGLYCAEMIC EMERGENCIES

In this chapter the diagnosis, management and prevention of hypoglycaemia and the hyperglycaemic emergencies will be discussed. Education of patients about the prevention of these conditions and early diagnosis are essential because coma due to both hyper- and hypoglycaemia is usually avoidable.

■ Hypoglycaemia

Hypoglycaemia is the commonest cause of loss of consciousness in diabetic patients, and of all the complications of diabetes, it is the one that patients fear most. It usually occurs in insulin treated patients but can also affect patients treated with a sulphonylurea. Because the manifestations are due to the rate of fall of blood glucose as well as the actual level, it is difficult to define a level of blood glucose that constitutes the boundary between normal and low levels. Insulin treated patients who maintain strict diabetic control may be able to tolerate lower levels of blood glucose without developing symptoms than a patient who maintains higher blood glucose concentrations. Although there may be a marked difference in hypogly-caemic symptoms between different patients, the symptoms tend to be relatively constant within the same patient.

The clinical features are caused by an overactivity of the sympathetic nervous system and a depressed activity of the central nervous system (Table 1). Some of the typical symptoms may be masked by certain drugs (e.g. beta-blockers, alcohol) or if the patient has autonomic neuropathy. Moreover, with increasing duration of diabetes some patients lose their awareness of hypoglycaemic symptoms. It is particularly important to teach family members how to recognise hypoglycaemia in such cases.

59

TABLE 1 MANIFESTATIONS OF HYPOGLYCAEMIA

Adrenergic	Neuroglycopenic
Sweating	Headache
Palpitations	Confusion
Tremor	Visual disturbances
Nervousness	Amnesia
Irritability	Seizure
Hunger	Focal signs, e.g. hemiplegia
Tachycardia	Coma

The commonest causes of hypoglycaemia are:

- Taking more exercise than usual
- Delay or omission of a snack or main meal
- Administration of too much insulin
- Eating insufficient carbohydrate
- Over-indulgence in alcohol
- A change from beef or pork to human insulin without a reduction in dosage
- Mistake in sulphonylurea dosage

Every insulin treated patient and their relatives should be taught the following:

1. The commonest causes of hypoglycaemia and, as prevention is better than treatment, they should know how to tackle the problem.
2. The recognition of signs and symptoms of hypoglycaemia and how to treat them.
3. Hypoglycaemia sometimes progresses very rapidly. Therefore, always carry sugar on your person and in your car; stop what you are doing and start treatment as soon as symptoms appear.
4. Always carry some form of identification stating that you have diabetes and should be given sugar if you are found ill.

In addition, most insulin treated patients and their relatives should know how to use glucagon.

Treatment of hypoglycaemia

Mild reactions
Most cases are mild and are treated by the patient or a family member. Twenty grams of rapidly absorbed carbohydrate, e.g. four glucose tablets or sugar lumps, is usually adequate but may need to be repeated if the symptoms have not resolved after 5–10 minutes. If the next meal or snack is not due for some time it is sensible to take some more slowly absorbed carbohydrate, e.g. an apple or a slice of bread, after recovery.

Severe reactions
Severe hypoglycaemia may cause stupor, coma, fits or focal neurological signs such as a hemiparesis. If hypoglycaemia is suspected a fingerprick blood sample should be obtained for estimation of blood glucose concentration using a blood glucose monitoring strip. If no means of estimating the blood glucose is available a therapeutic trial of intramuscular glucagon (1 mg) or intravenous dextrose should be given. The usual intravenous dose for an adult is 50 ml of 50 % dextrose given into an antecubital vein. Extravascular injection of dextrose may cause a painful thrombophlebitis, and if the patient is agitated or restless 1 mg of glucagon intramuscularly is preferable. Following recovery the patient should be given 30 g of slowly absorbed carbohydrate orally if the next meal is not immediately due.

Indications for hospital admission include poor or incomplete recovery from severe hypoglycaemia, recurrent severe reactions, or poor home circumstances such as an elderly patient living alone who has a severe reaction for no obvious reason.

Recurrent hypoglycaemia

There are a number of possible causes of recurrent episodes of hypoglycaemia.

1. *Altered patterns of eating or exercise*
   This is often associated with a change in employment which may involve more physical exercise or altered times for meal breaks. Consider the possibility of anorexia or bulimia nervosa, especially in younger women.

2. *Reduced insulin requirements*
   The commonest cause is a change from beef or pork to human insulin.

Weight loss of any cause is often associated with a reduction in insulin or oral hypoglycaemic requirements, as is the onset of renal failure. A dramatic reduction in insulin dosage is sometimes needed in the first few months after diagnosis of Type I diabetes — the so-called 'honeymoon' period.

3. *Altered awareness of hypoglycaemia*
Some patients find that they get less warning of the onset of hypoglycaemia after changing from beef or pork to human insulin. Other causes of altered awareness include the onset of autonomic neuropathy or treatment with beta-blockers.

4. *Alcohol abuse*
Alcohol abuse may cause recurrent attacks of hypoglycaemia (see Chapter 12).

5. *Other drug therapy*
This may potentiate the effects of oral hypoglycaemics (see Chapter 5, Table 3).

6. *Giving too much insulin*
Although this may seem obvious, it may be overlooked and a careful history should be taken.

The management of recurrent hypoglycaemia requires:

1. Assessment of the following aspects of insulin administration.
   i.   Injection sites should be carefully checked since lipohypertrophy can alter the rate of absorption.
   ii. Injection techniques must be checked since intradermal instead of subcutaneous injections may affect absorption.
   iii. It should also be remembered that hot baths and sun bathing can alter skin temperature and speed up absorption of insulin.
   iv. It is important to ensure that the patient's eyesight permits them to see accurately the markings on the syringe.
2. Enquiry into altered patterns of eating or exercise, and alcohol consumption. The type of insulin should be considered, e.g. a patient on beef lente may have been given

human lente inadvertently. Other drug therapy should also be reviewed and changes in body weight or renal function should be noted.

3. Inappropriate eating patterns, e.g. omission of a mid-morning snack leading to pre-lunch hypoglycaemia, should be corrected.

4. The dosage of insulin or oral hypoglycaemic agent should then be reduced if appropriate.

Nocturnal hypoglycaemia

The patient or his relatives may be woken by symptoms which occur at the time of the hypoglycaemic episode, but sometimes the only clues to the occurrence of nocturnal hypoglycaemia may be symptoms which occur some hours later when the patient awakes. Such symptoms include morning headaches, dizziness, forgetfulness, and confusion. Daytime sweats occurring in the absence of hypoglycaemia can sometimes follow an episode of nocturnal hypoglycaemia. A history of night sweats or of nocturnal fits should prompt consideration of night time hypos as a possible cause.

The blood glucose concentration on waking may be normal or even high. The finding of a high blood glucose concentration on waking does not exclude the possibility of nocturnal hypoglycaemia, which most commonly occurs between 2 and 4 a.m. If the diagnosis is suspected the patient should be asked to set his alarm clock for 2 a.m. on one occasion and 4 a.m. on another so that a fingerprick blood glucose can be checked at those times. The management is that described under 'Recurrent hypoglycaemia' above.

Hypoglycaemia caused by sulphonylureas

Hypoglycaemic reactions may occur in tablet-treated patients, and are most often seen during treatment with chlorpropamide and glibenclamide (see Chapter 5). Although patients respond to treatment with glucose, the half-life of these drugs is longer than most insulins, and recurrent hypoglycaemia may follow the initial reaction. Hospitalisation is often required with severe reactions. After recovery, the need for any treatment other than diet should be questioned but, if treatment with a sulphonylurea is deemed necessary, other drugs such as gliclazide or tolbutamide may be prescribed. Alternatively, metformin, which does not cause hypoglycaemia, may be prescribed if appropriate.

■ Hyperglycaemic emergencies

Diabetic ketoacidosis (DKA) and **hyperosmolar, non-ketotic hyperglycaemia** are life threatening conditions which should usually be preventable. The evolution of hyperglycaemic emergencies is less dramatic than the onset of hypoglycaemia, with the symptoms developing over hours or even days. Early intervention can therefore prevent the need for hospital referral, but **once the conditions are established immediate admission is mandatory**. The term 'coma' is best avoided in the nomenclature of these conditions because most patients are not comatose.

During stressful situations many patients experience transient deterioration of glycaemic control that may necessitate alteration to therapy. Events such as intercurrent illnesses, psychological stresses, the prescription of medication (e.g. steroids, diuretics; see also Chapter 13 and Appendix 3) or even menstruation (Chapter 11) may be associated with increased insulin requirements. Other causes of hyperglycaemia in a previously well-controlled patient include dietary indiscretion, reduction in physical activity and incorrect doses of either insulin or OHGs. Identification of the cause and a temporary increase in insulin or OHG dosage may prevent the development of a hyperglycaemic emergency (see also Chapter 15).

Diabetic ketoacidosis

DKA results from an absolute or relative deficiency of insulin leading to increased production and decreased utilisation of glucose, followed by catabolism of fat and protein. Rapid catabolism of fat results in synthesis of ketone bodies which cause the acidosis. Severe dehydration is common.

The common causes

1. Infections or other acute illnesses which cause increased output of counter-regulatory hormones (catecholamines, cortisol, glucagon). A normal individual would respond by increasing his endogenous insulin production, but this is impossible in Type I diabetic patients.
2. Omission of insulin or reduction in insulin dosage. Patients who are anorexic or vomiting sometimes mistakenly reduce the dose of insulin or stop it altogether, fearing that insulin will cause hypoglycaemia if they are unable to eat but, as explained in the preceding paragraph, it is more likely that the stress associated with the illness will require an increased insulin dosage.

Patients (and their doctors) must know:
- NEVER STOP INSULIN
- Test more frequently and increase the insulin dose if blood or urine glucose is high
- Seek URGENT medical help if a high glucose concentration does not rapidly respond to an increased dose of insulin, or there is more than a trace of ketonuria (for example see Case 1 below)

Symptoms of DKA result from:
- Hyperglycaemia — thirst and polyuria
- Acidosis — nausea, vomiting, hyperventilation, lethargy and disturbance of consciousness

Indications for immediate hospital admission are:
1. Repeated vomiting or inability take adequate oral fluids
2. Hyperventilation
3. Any disturbance of consciousness
4. Persistent ketonuria of more than a 'trace' on ketostix testing

Less severe cases may also require admission depending on social circumstances or other illness. DKA can deteriorate very rapidly — **if in doubt, admit**.

The following case histories illustrate differences between mild hyperglycaemia, which can be safely managed at home, and a severe case requiring immediate hospital admission:

Case 1

A 46 year old woman with longstanding Type I diabetes requests a visit from her GP because of an infective exacerbation of her chronic obstructive airways disease. She states that she has lowered her twice daily soluble and isophane insulin doses as her appetite is reduced but, despite eating little, she noticed increased thirst and intermittent ketonuria. There are no abnormal signs on examination but she has a pyrexia and a cough productive of green sputum. A blood glucose is 21 mmol/l and urinalysis shows 1 + ketones and 4 +

glucose. Ampicillin is prescribed for her infection and an increase in insulin dosage is advised, despite her reduced appetite. She is also advised to monitor her blood glucose at least every four hours and, if necessary, to further increase her insulin according to the results. Dietary advice is given as suggested on page 155. Two days later she is feeling better, with results of HBGM of less than 11 mmol/l and an increased appetite.

Comment: This patient had developed hyperglycaemia as a result of a chest infection and this problem had been exacerbated because she had incorrectly lowered her insulin dosage when ill. All Type I diabetic patients must be taught that insulin requirements are usually increased during illness even if the appetite is reduced. With treatment of the chest infection, together with an increase in insulin doses she made a satisfactory recovery without hospital admission.

Case 2

A 21 year old male student with a three year history of Type I diabetes returns from a holiday on the Continent and presents with a two day history of nausea, vomiting and diarrhoea. Despite increasing his insulin doses, blood glucose results remain high and he is unable to eat or drink because of persistent vomiting. On examination he appears dyspnoeic and dehydrated, blood glucose 29 mmol/l; urine: 4 + glucose, 3 + ketones.

Urgent hospital referral is indicated here as a diagnosis of DKA is likely.

Hyperosmolar non-ketotic hyperglycaemia

The main features of this less common condition, which tends to affect elderly and West Indian patients, are hyperglycaemia and dehydration. The patient, often with tablet treated Type II diabetes, develops severe hyperglycaemia with associated thirst which may be neglected or fuelled by drinking beverages with a high sugar content such as Lucozade. Disturbances in consciousness often occur in this condition which has a high mortality. The blood glucose concentration is markedly elevated, though ketonuria may be absent or minimal. **Any patient suspected of having this condition should be referred to hospital as a matter of urgency**. The dehydration is often very severe and secondary thrombotic events are common.

Finally, remember that other non-diabetic causes of a disturbed conscious level or coma occur in diabetic patients just as frequently, if not more frequently than in non-diabetic individuals.

Further reading

Hypoglycaemia

Gill G.V. and Alberti K.G.G.M. (1985). *Practical Diabetes* 2(5), 5–10.

Diabetes ketoacidosis

Gill G.V. and Alberti K.G.G.M. (1985). *Practical Diabetes* 2(1), 15–20.

Hyperosmolar non-ketotic hyperglycaemia

Gill G.V. and Alberti K.G.G.M. (1985). *Practical Diabetes* 2(3), 30–35.

8 | CHRONIC COMPLICATIONS

The prevalence of long-term complications is thought to be related to the duration of diabetes, the quality of diabetic control, and probably also to genetic and environmental influences which are, as yet, poorly understood.

These complications are of insidious onset and irreversible by the time that they cause symptoms. However, their progression may be arrested or slowed if they are recognised sufficiently early. It is therefore important that patients be taught about these complications and the steps which they can take to minimise the consequences. It is equally important that every patient should have an annual review examination (see Chapter 16), so that complications are detected at the earliest possible time.

■ The painful diabetic leg

Both **peripheral neuropathy** and **vascular disease** are common complications of diabetes, their prevalence increasing with age and duration of disease. It is important to distinguish neuropathic from vascular pain in the leg because the management is different. Suggestive symptoms and signs of each condition are listed in Table 1, though neuropathic and vascular symptoms often co-exist.

Neuropathy

Distal sensory neuropathy
This is the commonest of the diabetic neuropathies. Patients usually present with a gradual onset of paraesthetic and painful symptoms in the lower limbs (Table 1). These symptoms are typically characterised by nocturnal exacerbation, with bedclothes irritating the hyperaesthetic skin. The sensory symptoms may lead to a curious sensation when walking that has been likened to 'walking on air' or 'walking on pillows'. A particularly

TABLE 1 COMMON SYMPTOMS AND SIGNS OF PERIPHERAL
NEUROPATHY AND VASCULAR DISEASE

Neuropathy	Vascular
Paraesthesiae, numbness	Intermittent claudication
Burning/shooting pain	Rest pain (different character to
Hyperaesthesiae	neuropathic pain)
Loss of temperature/vibration	Reduced/absent foot pulses
perception	Arterial bruits
Small muscle wasting in feet	Pallor on foot elevation
Reduced/absent tendon reflexes	Cool feet

TABLE 2 SOME CAUSES OF NEUROPATHY

- Diabetes*
- Malignancy*
- Renal failure*
- Drugs*
- Alcohol*
- Toxins
- B12 Deficiency
- Thiamine Deficiency
- Hereditary Neuropathies

* More common causes.

dangerous situation is that described as the 'painful–painless leg', in which
the patient experiences painful symptoms, but has reduced pain sensation
on examination: such patients are at great risk of painless injury to their
feet.

Examination usually reveals patchy sensory loss in a stocking and glove
distribution. However some patients develop symptoms before there is any
definite abnormality on clinical examination.

The differential diagnosis is from other causes of a peripheral neuropathy
(Table 2).

Treatment is summarised in Table 3. Poor glycaemic control should be
corrected if possible, although improved control does not always benefit
neuropathic symptoms. There is some evidence that painful neuropathy is
more common in those who drink more than 20 units of alcohol weekly, and

TABLE 3 TREATMENT OF SYMPTOMATIC PERIPHERAL NEURO-PATHY
1. Improve glycaemic control, if appropriate and feasible
2. Reduce alcohol consumption to less than 20 units per week
3. Bed cradle if nocturnal symptoms
4. If symptoms persist, try simple analgesics
5. If no benefit, try imipramine 25–75 mg nocte
6. If no improvement after 2–3 weeks, try carbamazepine or phenytoin
7. Avoid narcotic analgesics

a decrease in consumption may help. A bed cradle to lift the bedclothes off sensitive feet is often remarkably effective. If simple analgesics do not help, a tricyclic drug such as imipramine should be tried: the mode of action is on the peripheral nerves rather than simply treating any associated insomnia or depression.

The prognosis depends upon a number of factors: the younger patient with acute sensory symptoms but few signs has a favourable outlook, whereas the insidious onset of symptoms and signs in an older patient suggests a longer course. Improvement in symptoms is not necessarily a favourable sign: the patient may be left with an insensitive foot which is at risk of ulceration.

Proximal motor neuropathy ('amyotrophy')
Proximal motor neuropathy is much less common than a distal sensory neuropathy. Patients, who are often men over 60 years old, present with pain in the thighs, weakness and wasting which is often asymmetrical, and difficulty walking. The main differential diagnoses are carcinomatous neuropathy or spinal cord disorders. Treatment is that described for sensory neuropathy together with intensive physiotherapy.

Vascular pain

A history of **claudication** with absent foot pulses on examination is the commonest presentation. Nocturnal **rest pain** indicates more advanced vascular disease. It is typically relieved by hanging the feet over the edge of the bed and is aggravated by walking, whereas nocturnal neuropathic pain is relieved by walking.

> **The principles of management** are the same as in a non-diabetic patient, namely:
> 1. Cessation of smoking
> 2. Aim for a normal body weight
> 3. Withdraw beta-blocking drugs if possible

There is no place for vasodilator therapy which has not been shown to improve symptoms in carefully controlled trials. The patient with a stable claudicating distance should be encouraged to exercise.

> **Indications for hospital referral include:**
> ● worsening claudication
> ● rest pain
> ● ischaemic lesions on the feet
> ● any foot ulcer associated with vascular insufficiency

The increasing availability of angioplasty has meant that many patients who are unfit for major vascular surgery can now be treated. Finally, as most patients have an associated autonomic neuropathy, there is virtually no indication for the procedure of lumbar sympathectomy in the management of diabetic peripheral vascular disease.

■ Diabetic foot problems

Foot problems are a major cause of morbidity and an occasional cause of death in diabetic patients. Diabetic patients spend more days in hospital with foot diseases than they do for any other cause, **yet these problems are frequently preventable**.

Patients most at risk

Of the risk factors listed in Table 4 the most important are peripheral neuropathy and peripheral vascular disease. The patient with reduced pain sensation often subjects his feet to abnormally high pressures, temperatures or other traumas because he feels no discomfort. Such patients may present with large, painless ulcers. A patient with a foot ulcer who walks without a limp almost certainly has neuropathy. The neuropathic foot may feel warm and may appear superficially healthy but is at great risk of ulceration.

TABLE 4 PATIENTS MOST AT RISK OF FOOT PROBLEMS

Peripheral neuropathy
Peripheral vascular disease
Previous foot problems
Deformity of feet
  e.g. claw toes, hallux valgus
Other diabetic complications
  e.g. retinopathy, especially if associated with visual handicap
Obesity
Elderly patients, especially those
  incapable of caring for themselves

Patients who are overweight inevitably subject their feet to greater pressures than do those of normal weight.

Prevention

Screening
The aim of screening is to detect those patients who are at risk so that preventative measures can be instituted. Surveys have shown that only a

TABLE 5 CHECKLIST FOR FOOT EXAMINATION

Danger signs	Thick callus In-growing toe nails Local erythema/tenderness Skin breaks (check between toes)
Sensory	Vibration, pain and proprioceptive sensation
Motor	Wasting, weakness, absent ankle reflex
Autonomic	Dry warm skin
Vascular	Foot pulses, skin temperature, pallor
Shape	Toe deformities (e.g. clawing, hammer toes), hallux valgus, prominent metatarsal heads, Charcot deformity

small proportion of doctors regularly examine the feet of their diabetic patients. If we do not set an example by showing interest in the problem, we should not be surprised if our patients ignore advice about foot care. **All patients should have a regular foot examination,** ideally once a year at their annual review. The components of the examination are listed in Table 5. Assessment of vibration perception is one of the most useful tests and any patient who is unable to feel the vibration of a 128 tuning fork in the feet should be considered at great risk.

Those patients with risk factors should be given specific advice about foot care and referred, if necessary, to the chiropodist or diabetes clinic.

Those patients without risk factors should be advised, in more general terms, of the possibility of foot problems occurring at a later date and advised to maintain a high standard of foot hygiene.

TABLE 6 ADVICE TO PATIENTS AT RISK OF FOOT ULCER

DO	DO NOT
• Inspect feet daily, using a mirror if necessary to see the underneath of the foot	• Walk barefoot
	• Smoke
• Wash feet daily using warm (not hot) water	• Step into bath without checking temperature
• Apply lotion/oil to feet if the skin is dry	• Use hot water bottles
• Avoid extremes of temperature	• Use corn plasters or try to cut your own corns
• Have your feet checked at clinic visits	• Use pummice stones, nail files or chemicals to remove hard skin
• Inspect shoes daily for nails, etc	• Wear new shoes for more than an hour or two at a time
• Attend chiropodist regularly if advised to do so	
• Seek help promptly if a lesion appears	

Education
Teaching patients about foot care has been shown to reduce the frequency of major amputations. The advice which should be given to 'at risk' patients is summarised in Table 6. Several pharmaceutical companies supply useful leaflets about diabetic foot care and educational videotapes on this subject have been produced by Servier Laboratories, Lipha Pharmaceuticals and the British Diabetic Association.

Chiropody
The chiropodist not only deals with toe nails, corns and callus but can often also provide simple orthoses to help prevent foot disorders, as well as reinforcing advice given by doctors and nurses.

Shoes
Unsuitable footwear can cause problems which result in amputations in diabetic patients, and good, well designed shoes can prevent ulceration and amputation. 'At risk' patients should be considered for referral to the shoe fitter. The essential points in the design of a diabetic shoe are:

1. It should be of a sufficiently broad fitting, and with adequate depth to accommodate claw-toes if present.
2. Uppers should be constructed of soft leather with no toe-puffs or other stiffening.
3. High heels, which throw excessive weight onto the forefoot, should be avoided.
4. Insoles must be cushioned with a material which is soft enough to absorb shocks but not so soft that it 'bottoms out'.
5. A rigid cradle to redistribute weight may be needed under the insole.

Foam troughs
Foam troughs are essential equipment for the at-risk patient who is confined to bed, whether he is in hospital or at home. The trough is placed under the leg with the foot protruding beyond the end of the trough so that vulnerable heels are protected from pressure.

Management of established foot problems

The patient with an established problem is best referred to a hospital clinic for initial diagnosis and advice on management, even if subsequent care is provided by the general practitioner and community nurse. Only in the hospital clinic is the combined expertise of doctor, chiropodist and shoe fitter readily available.

■ Diabetic eye disease

Diabetic retinopathy

Diabetic retinopathy is the commonest cause of blindness in people of working age in this country. **Regular screening for early signs of retinopathy is essential** because blindness is preventable if treatment is given at an early stage but symptoms may not develop until the condition is well advanced.

Risk factors

The prevalence of retinopathy is related to:

1. Increasing duration of diabetes.
2. Age at diagnosis: 25% of patients aged 40 and over will have retinopathy within 10 years, but only 7% of those aged less than 20 at diagnosis will develop retinopathy within 10 years.
3. Poor glycaemic control (although some patients with good control will develop retinopathy).
4. The presence of other microvascular complications, e.g. proteinuria or neuropathy.
5. Hypertension, and possibly also
6. Cigarette smoking.

In addition, established retinopathy may deteriorate during pregnancy.

Frequency of screening

If possible, those patients who are attending for their annual review should have their records marked so that the clinic staff know to dilate the pupils upon arrival.

There has recently been much debate on the subject of who should screen the fundi. Although the opticians frequently examine the patients' eyes, the ultimate diagnosis of retinopathy does rest upon the medical staff and, in our view, screening should be performed regularly by either mini-clinic staff or the hospital diabetes clinic even if the patients are also attending an optician regularly.

Types of retinopathy

The main types of retinopathy are shown in Table 7. Publications containing colour plates of diabetic retinopathy are listed under 'Further reading' at the end of the chapter. A careful examination of the entire retina is required, remembering that new vessels may first occur peripherally. The presence of any pre-proliferative or proliferative changes should lead to an

TABLE 7 A CLASSIFICATION OF DIABETIC RETINOPATHY

Type	Features	Action
Background	Microaneurysms (dots) Retinal haemorrhages (blots) Retinal vein dilatation Hard exudates	Review annually Refer if visual acuity impaired or if more than just a few scattered exudates
Maculopathy	Macular oedema Macular exudates and haemorrhages	Refer to ophthalmologist for early appointment (within one month)
Pre-proliferative	Cotton wool spots (soft 'exudates') Venous beading Arteriolar sheathing	As above
Proliferative	New vessels Pre-retinal haemorrhages Vitreous haemorrhages	Patients with new vessels should be seen by an ophthalmologist within two weeks. Pre-retinal or vitreous haemorrhage requires immediate referral by telephone
Advanced	Fibrous proliferation ± traction retinal detachment	Early referral for consideration of vitrectomy to prevent retinal detachment

In all cases consider whether glycaemic control can be improved and look for hypertension or other risk factors which can be corrected.

urgent referral to the ophthalmologist. In addition, those with signs of maculopathy (see Table 7) also require referral. Many diabetic and ophthalmological clinics welcome general practitioners who wish to increase their expertise of fundoscopy. Macular oedema and fine new vessels can be difficult for the less experienced observer to recognise. The presence of macular oedema may be suggested by impairment of visual acuity, even when corrected by a pinhole, without any other obvious cause such as cataracts.

The diagnosis of retinopathy may require referral to an ophthalmologist (see Table 7) and should always lead to a review of the adequacy of glycaemic control and a check for correctable risk factors such as hypertension.

Examining the eyes

1. *Test the visual acuity*
   Test each eye separately using a Snellen chart. If the patient wears glasses for distant vision, these should be worn. If the visual acuity is still worse than 6/6, correct for any refractive error by using a pinhole.

2. *Dilate the pupils*
   Tropicamide 0.5% is suitable for most patients. Reversal with pilocarpine is not necessary. Warn patients about blurred vision and that care must be taken if driving afterwards. **Narrow angle glaucoma and previous eye surgery are contra-indications**; these patients should be assessed by an ophthalmologist.

3. *Fundus examination*
   Good batteries in the ophthalmoscope are essential for an adequate view, and the examination should preferably be carried out in a darkened room. A good ophthalmoscope with which the examiner is familiar should be used. Look first for evidence of cataract and then focus on the retina, examining the optic disc, and then make a careful examination of the peripheral retina and finally the macula.

Other eye conditions associated with diabetes

Refractive errors
Refractive errors due to hyperglycaemia are common, particularly following correction of hyperglycaemia after diagnosis. Patients should be advised to delay visiting an optician for new spectacles until the diabetes has been stabilised for a month.

Cataracts
These are more common in diabetic patients and tend to occur at a younger age. Patients should be referred if there is significant impairment of visual acuity, or if the cataract prevents an adequate examination of the retina.

Vitreous haemorrhage and retinal detachment
These may be a late consequence of proliferative diabetic retinopathy. Patients with these conditions require an urgent ophthalmological referral.

Retinal vein occlusion
This can be associated with diabetes, hypertension or any cause of a raised blood viscosity. Immediate referral is required because treatment may prevent subsequent new vessel formation.

Rubeosis of the iris
Rubeosis is a pink discoloration of the iris due to new blood vessels growing on the surface of the iris. It may result in glaucoma, and urgent referral is indicated.

Cranial nerve palsies
These may occur in diabetes. Exclusion of more sinister causes is essential and prompt referral indicated.

The role of the ophthalmologist

When a patient is referred for assessment, a fluorescein angiogram is quite commonly requested. This is an outpatient procedure that is used to demonstrate abnormalities of the vascular architecture of the fundus.

The commonest treatment of diabetic retinopathy is laser beam photo-coagulation which is usually performed as an outpatient procedure. Indications for this therapy would include the presence of proliferative retinopathy or maculopathy. For some patients with advanced diabetic retinopathy often associated with retinal detachment, vitrectomy surgery may be performed and this requires a general anaesthetic and an inpatient stay of about seven days.

■ Diabetic nephropathy

Nephropathy will eventually develop in 20–40% of Type I diabetic patients and, from the onset of proteinuria, will typically progress to end stage renal disease (ESRD) in an average of 11 years. Diabetic nephropathy now accounts for a quarter of patients entering the end stage renal disease programmes in the UK. Although most research into the natural history of this condition has been in Type I diabetes, nephropathy also complicates Type II diabetes in which it is associated with an increase in morbidity and mortality from vascular causes.

Risk factors

Those who are at particular risk of nephropathy are patients with Type I diabetes of greater than 10 years' duration (especially if they also have retinopathy), or any patients with Type II diabetes and retinopathy, especially if hypertensive.

Definitions

Diabetic nephropathy
A clinical diagnosis made when persistent albustix-positive proteinuria develops in a diabetic patient with no other apparent cause of proteinuria. It is the clinical manifestation of the pathological lesion, diabetic glomerulosclerosis.

Microalbuminuria
The presence of an increased albumin excretion in an albustix-negative patient. It is an early marker for diabetic nephropathy, and is likely to become more widely available as a screening test for nephropathy in future years.

End stage renal disease (ESRD)
Advanced renal failure necessitating dialysis or transplantation.

Natural history

The onset of diabetic nephropathy is gradual and will only be detected if the urine is regularly tested for protein. As with retinopathy, symptoms only appear when the condition is at an advanced stage, with severe deterioration of renal function. Proteinuria is usually intermittent initially, but subsequently the protein loss becomes continuous and increases slowly over years. The serum creatinine concentration is initially normal but, as the associated hypertension develops, a gradual reduction in glomerular filtration rate follows. If the proteinuria and hypertension remain undetected, the first symptoms may be due to fluid retention (ankle oedema, breathlessness) or uraemia.

TABLE 8 INVESTIGATION OF PERSISTENT OR INTERMITTENT PROTEINURIA

1. Check BP and look for retinopathy
2. Send MSU for culture to exclude infection
3. Check renal function tests, serum albumin and 24 hour urine for protein excretion
4. Consider hospital referral

Proteinuria is the first sign of nephropathy and all patients should have an annual urine test for protein. Impairment of renal function in the absence of either proteinuria or retinopathy suggests that the renal condition is not due to the diabetes.

If proteinuria is detected on a dipstick investigation the test should be repeated, preferably on an early morning sample. A regular finding of proteinuria, even if intermittent, requires further investigation (Table 8). Hospital referral should be considered to confirm the diagnosis of diabetic nephropathy.

Management

Hypertension
Hypertension (see Chapter 13) should be treated aggressively because this has been shown to slow the progression of nephropathy. The aim should be to achieve a normal, or near normal, blood pressure in younger patients and a systolic of less than 160 mmHg in older patients.

Protein restriction
Protein restriction with emphasis on vegetables as the main source of dietary protein may also slow the rate at which nephropathy advances.

Good glycaemic control
This should be established if possible, particularly in early stages of nephropathy. There is no evidence that good glycaemic control will have any useful effect on established nephropathy but it may benefit any associated retinopathy.

The **renal threshold for glucose** may be altered in nephropathy and urine tests are an unreliable means of assessing control. Measurements of **glycosylated haemoglobin** may be spuriously high in uraemic patients because some assays also measure carbamylated haemoglobin.

Insulin requirements

Insulin requirements may decrease as renal function deteriorates. Patients with Type II diabetes and impaired glomerular function should **not** be given **metformin**, and short acting **sulphonylureas** are usually preferable to long acting drugs such as chlorpropamide (Chapter 5).

Management of end stage renal disease

Diabetic patients are now more likely to receive treatment for ESRD than they were a few years ago. Most are now treated initially with chronic ambulatory peritoneal dialysis, but the treatment of choice is transplantation with a well matched donor kidney. Haemodialysis is rarely used as a long-term treatment because of problems with vascular access in diabetes and because the risk of blindness from retinal haemorrhage is increased.

■ Some other chronic complications

Lipoatrophy and lipohypertrophy

These terms refer to atrophy or hypertrophy of the subcutaneous tissues at the site of insulin injections. Lipoatrophy typically occurs in children or young women soon after diagnosis. It was more common with the older, less pure beef insulins than with the recently introduced monocomponent pork or human insulins. Both conditions can be prevented or minimised by frequent rotation of injection sites.

Necrobiosis lipoidica

Lesions typically occur on the shins and consist of small red nodules or plaques which then flatten and develop a brown or yellow colour. The lesions can be unsightly and may ulcerate. Treatment requires referral to a specialist for consideration of topical or intra-lesional steroid, but the results are often disappointing.

Occasionally necrobiosis precedes the diagnosis of diabetes and the patient presenting with such lesions should always be screened to exclude hyperglycaemia.

Cheiroarthopathy

Some patients develop thickening and tightness of the skin and underlying connective tissue with flexion contractures of the small joints of the hands. It is rarely severe enough to cause any functional disability. It is still uncertain whether it is associated with poor glycaemic control and other chronic complications such as retinopathy.

■ Further reading

Diabetic foot disease

Bell P.R.F. (1983). Assessment of peripheral vascular disease. *Practical Diabetes* **3**, 203–204.

Edmonds M.E. (1984; 1985). The diabetic foot. *Practical Diabetes* **1**; **2** (5 articles).

Foster A. and Edmonds M.E. (1987). Examination of the diabetic foot. *Practical Diabetes* **4**, 105–106; 153–154.

Tovey F.I. (1986). Care of the diabetic foot. *Practical Diabetes* **3**, 130–134.

Diabetic eye disease

Kohner E.M. *et al.* (1985; 1986) Seven articles on diabetic eye disease. *Practical Diabetes*, **2**; **3**.

Kritzinger E.E. and Taylor K.G. *Diabetic Eye Disease: an Illustrated Guide to Diagnosis and Management.* MTP Press Ltd., Lancaster. 1984, 88 pp. This short manual is essential reading for anyone examining diabetic eyes.

Manifestations of Sight-Threatening Retinopathy. An 18-page photographic reference manual contained in the RCGP folder on *Diabetes* and also available from DLB Systems Ltd., The Innovation Centre, Cambridge Science Park, Cambridge CB4 4BG.

Diabetic nephropathy

Practical Diabetes, 1985, **2**(3), 12–28 (4 articles).

9 EDUCATION

Tis not knowing much but what is useful that makes man wise
Thomas Fuller, 1732

One of the most significant advances in diabetes in recent years has been the increased emphasis that has been placed on education of both patients and staff. Patients are now recognised as the most important members of the diabetes team: they seek basic advice from medical and nursing staff in order to achieve optimal control of their condition. Diabetes is almost unique amongst chronic medical conditions as the patients can monitor and treat their own illness, provided that they have a sound understanding of both the condition itself and its management. A lack of education and understanding of diabetes and its complications may have serious consequences: many unnecessary hospital admissions result from the failure of patients or medical staff to interpret correctly the symptoms, signs and blood glucose results during an acute illness. It has been estimated that at least half of all amputations in our patients are potentially preventable. Masson and colleagues (1989) recently reported that the majority of foot ulcer patients had no recollection of having previously received education about foot care, and had little idea of simple foot care including the need to have feet measured when buying shoes. Thus a simple, structured educational programme may prove to be one of the most important areas of patient management. However, it is essential to remember Fuller's words, to keep all educational material simple and succinct, and not to burden the patient with unnecessary information.

■ Medical education

Before embarking on diabetes education, it is vital that medical and nursing staff have a sound knowledge of diabetes and its complications. Many postgraduate medical education centres run courses on diabetes and recent experience has shown that these are extremely well attended. A national advanced postgraduate course is held each January, and is hosted by the University of Newcastle Upon Tyne until 1992: this is primarily for career diabetologists though many GP clinical assistants have attended in previous years. A similar course specifically for GPs is currently at the planning stage.

The diabetes specialist nurses and practice nurses are often responsible for patient education, and you should consider sending your practice nurse on the English National Board Course 928 (ENB 928) entitled *Diabetic Nursing for Registered Nurses and Midwives*. This course is now held in many nursing schools throughout the country.

■ Patient education

It is essential before embarking upon any educational programme to have the aims and objectives clearly defined. Although patients inevitably vary enormously in intelligence, educational background, age, motivation, and so on, it is still advisable to have a **check list** of educational aims which can be ticked off as each item is covered. The overall aims of such a programme should be: (a) to help the patient accept the diagnosis, (b) to help the patient understand about diabetes, its treatment, potential complications and day-to-day management, and (c) to continually motivate the patient.

Before outlining the areas that should be covered in any particular course of patient education, it is important to state certain principles.

1. The members of the diabetes team must identify and agree upon the educational priorities before starting the course. What information is essential and what is not? What should be taught first, and what can be left until later?
2. The educational programme must allow time to establish or modify patient behaviour: there is little point in trying to teach everything immediately after diagnosis as the patient is often numbed or emotionally shocked and is unable to absorb any additional information. However, some points must be mentioned at the time of diagnosis such as advice on informing the DVLC, how to recognise hypos for those on insulin, and so on. Any information which is given soon after the patient has been told the diagnosis should be repeated at a later date.
3. All members of the team must preach the same message. In this regard, it is not unknown for contradictory advice to be given by colleagues and this simply confuses the patient.
4. Regular reinforcement and evaluation is necessary.
5. The educators must display optimism and have a firm belief that

adopting the way of life outlined in the programme will promote good health and reduce the chances of both short- and long-term complications developing.

The steps in the process of education may be summarised as follows:

- **Motivation:** it is the task of all those who come into contact with patients to motivate and encourage the patient in the management of their condition. In the community this includes the doctor, practice nurse, dietitian and chiropodist
- **Reception** of information
- **Application** of acquired knowledge to day-to-day diabetes management

Educational methods

Several methods of presentation may be used to provide the necessary information.

The spoken word

This includes lectures, group teaching, small group discussion and face-to-face tutorials. The individual consultation should always be used to provide information and this utilises the last method. The other techniques may be used, but require time and resources. It must be remembered that many patients hear what is presented, but only a few actually listen and register the information (to hear and forget!). Numerous studies have confirmed that newly-diagnosed patients forget most of that which they are told soon after diagnosis.

Using audio visual aids

The use of tape-slide presentations, films, computer-aided programmes and video-cassettes is becoming increasingly popular. Many educational videos are now available either free of charge or for a nominal cost: these can be used in conjunction with other teaching methods, or loaned to the patients who can then view them together with their families at home.

Using the written word

Leaflets and booklets that cover all aspects of diabetes, its management and complications are available from the British Diabetic Association and many of the major pharmaceutical houses in the diabetes area. There is a danger of stocking a variety of leaflets which cover similar areas but contain contradictory advice. It is, therefore, advisable to check all the literature that is available to the patient in the surgery to ensure that such a circumstance does not occur.

It is difficult to state which educational method gives the best results as so many variables exist. However, many centres succeed with a combination of the above techniques. One example is the use of a video to stimulate discussion in a small-group discussion situation, which is becoming increasingly popular. The practice nurse might be encouraged to form and lead such a group, which may also use educational literature to reinforce the message.

■ Course content

The precise content of an educational course for diabetic patients will depend on many factors including the age and intelligence of the patient, as well as their social, educational and racial background, in addition to the ideas of the doctors and nurses involved. However, most syllabuses would include the following eight topics.

What is diabetes?

This should be a short session and give a basic introduction to the condition. As this may be presented soon after the diagnosis, it must be restricted to essential information that is required in the first few weeks after diagnosis.

Healthy eating and diabetes

This is ideally presented by the community dietitian. The patient's relatives should be encouraged to attend as the advice on healthy eating usually applies to all!

Aims of diabetes treatment

This should include basic information on metabolic control and how this might be achieved.

Treatments

Depending on the type of diabetes, this should cover either oral hypoglycaemic agents or insulin types and methods of administration.

Monitoring

This should include urine monitoring for glucose or ketones, or home blood glucose monitoring, according to the needs of the patient.

Living with diabetes

This might include advice on the following:

● exercise
● work and diabetes
● driving
● problems with insurance
● other illnesses
● family planning

Acute complications

This is mainly for insulin treated patients and should cover hypoglycaemia together with hyperglycaemic emergencies. However, patients on sulphonylurea drugs must be informed about the possibility of hypoglycaemia occurring.

Chronic complications

Contrary to popular belief, most patients are soon aware that complications might occur and emphasis in this section should be on how these can be avoided. This will include the need for regular foot care, good glycaemic control and the avoidance of smoking. A basic knowledge of chronic complications helps the patient to understand the importance of attending for an annual review.

■ Ongoing education

The course outlined above refers to the beginning of what must be an ongoing process: revision, updating and reinforcement are essential components of the educational process. To this end, a number of useful courses are organised by the BDA, including:

● residential courses for adult patients
● family week-ends for those with diabetic children
● summer and educational holidays for children and adolescents (age 5–25)
● meetings organised by local BDA branches.

We must remember the words of Dr R.D. Lawrence — a founder member of the British Diabetic Association, and himself diabetic:

The diabetic patient must be his own doctor, dietitian, and laboratory technician. Hence education is the single most important aspect of treatment.

■ Teaching aids

The following aids are available from the British Diabetic Association, 10 Queen Anne Street, London, W1M OBD, either free of charge or for a nominal fee.

- *Introduction to Diabetes* — a leaflet
- *Introduction to Diabetes* — a tape/slide programme
- *Living with Diabetes* — short text by Dr Arnold Bloom
- *Diabetes Handbook* — by Dr John L. Day of Ipswich
  1. for patients with non-insulin dependent diabetes
  2. for patients with insulin dependent diabetes

Dietary teaching aids for lectures on diets — each contains 36 slides for £20 and are available for English or Ethnic diets. A number of leaflets on diets are also available. In addition, four cookery books may be purchased from the BDA. Teaching aids and books on all the other areas covered in this chapter are available from the BDA.

■ Education for self-monitoring

Urine testing

The instructions that come with the bottles are clear and really have to be read carefully and taught on a one-to-one basis with the patient.

Home blood glucose monitoring

The main companies in this area provide leaflets, audio visual aids and will arrange demonstrations for patients. **Contact addresses:** BCL Limited, Bell Lane, Lewes, East Sussex, BN7 1LG; Ames Corporation, Miles Laboratories Ltd., Ames Division, PO Box 37, Stoke Court, Stoke Poges, Slough, SL2 4LY; and Hypoguard UK Ltd., Dock Lane, Woodbridge, Suffolk, LP12 1PE.

Education for diabetes mini-clinics

The Royal College of General Practitioners produce a series of clinical information packs which is included in the diabetes folder. Any GP considering establishing a mini-clinic should purchase this very useful material. Servier Laboratories Ltd., Fulmer Hall, Windmill Road, Fulmer, Slough, SL3 6HH, provide a package for the diabetes mini-clinic which includes comprehensive documentation for the medical records and useful educational literature for the patients. In addition, Servier Laboratories will supply, free of charge (via the local representative) video cassettes for education of staff. These include videos on diabetic retinopathy and diabetic foot care for viewing by medical and nursing staff. Servier also provide another programme entitled *Staying on your Feet* for patients at risk of foot disease.

Other useful addresses are to be found in the appendices to this book.

Further reading

Baksi A.K., Hyde D.W. and Giles G. (Eds.) *Diabetes Education*. John Wiley, Chichester, 1984.

Day J.L. *Minimal Educational Facilities Report*. British Diabetic Association, London.

Hill R.D. Educating the diabetic. In: *Diabetes Health Care*, Chapman and Hall, London, 1987, pp. 21–36.

Masson E.A., Angle, S., Roseman, P. *et al.* (1989) Foot ulcers — do patients know how to protect themselves? *Practical Diabetes* **6**, 22–24.

10 LIVING WITH DIABETES

The patient with diabetes, particularly if treated with insulin, faces many problems in ordinary daily life. Doctors should be aware of these problems so that they can give appropriate advice. It is always sad to see youngsters who have, for example, set their hearts on a career in the army, and who get as far as applying before discovering that insulin treatment precludes their acceptance. A few words of explanation some years earlier could have avoided much disappointment.

■ Employment

Prejudice

The commonest problem is prejudice from employers. Such prejudice is usually born of ignorance and the belief that all people with diabetes have poor work records and that their work is regularly interrupted by attacks of hypoglycaemia. A letter of reference and explanation from a doctor can be very helpful. Some patients will try to conceal their diabetes from an employer. This should be discouraged as concealment can affect employment and pension rights. The insulin treated patient should also be encouraged to tell workmates about the symptoms and treatment of hypoglycaemia, so that they can take appropriate action if necessary.

Prohibited occupations

Certain occupations are not open to insulin treated patients (Table 1). There are other occupations which, although not prohibited, might be regarded as unsuitable for those on insulin, e.g. steeplejack, blast furnaceman.

Patients with Type II are usually also precluded from employment as airline pilots and may have restrictions placed on a passenger service

TABLE 1 PROHIBITED OR UNSUITABLE OCCUPATIONS FOR INSULIN TREATED PATIENTS

Usually prohibited	Unsuitable
Airline pilot	Steeplejack
Train driver	Blast furnaceman
Armed services	Etc.
Prison service	
Fire Brigade	
HGV ⎱ licence required PSV ⎰	
Professional diver, seaman	

vehicle (PSV) licence. Patients with Type II diabetes are not currently allowed to **join** the Armed Services, the Police, the Prison Service or the Fire brigade, but are usually allowed to drive mainline trains provided that they are not taking sulphonylureas. Serving seamen and oil rig workers with Type II diabetes are usually allowed to remain at sea subject to regular medical review.

Shift work can present problems but they are rarely insurmountable. Patients using insulin infusion pumps should have no problem, and those using the Novopen system can take their injection of long-acting Ultralente insulin before going to work instead of at bedtime. Advice given to patients who are on twice or once daily injections must be tailored to suit the individual's circumstances.

Irregular hours especially if associated with a variable physical workload present greater problems than regular shifts. The farmer who is up all night with a difficult calving will inevitably have more difficulty maintaining good control than the office worker with regular hours. As a general rule these patients are often best managed with small but frequent injections using a Novopen or, occasionally, with an infusion pump.

Careers guidance

School children should be aware of those occupations which are either prohibited or otherwise unsuitable, and should be encouraged to obtain the best possible academic qualifications so as to broaden the range of jobs which are open to them. Heavy manual work is not incompatible with good diabetic control but does make it more difficult to achieve. Older patients, especially those with diabetic complications, can sometimes find it advantageous to register as disabled in order to get appropriate work.

■ Sport and exercise

Sport and exercise appropriate to the age and general health of the individual should be encouraged as an integral part of a normal, healthy life, subject to the following considerations.

1. There are some sports where the participant is at the mercy of the weather and the elements or where hypoglycaemia could put other people's lives at risk (Table 2). These sports are best avoided by those on insulin.
2. Insulin treated patients with hyperglycaemia should avoid vigorous exercise until their blood glucose concentration is better controlled. Exertion may cause a rise in blood glucose concentration in insulin deficient patients, probably because the muscles are unable to use glucose which is released by the liver.
3. Patients with severe proliferative retinopathy should avoid vigorous exercise until the fragile new vessels have regressed following treatment, and patients with severe neuropathy should avoid prolonged running on hard surfaces.

Exercise and hypoglycaemia

Patients treated with insulin or sulphonylureas must be aware of the possibility of hypoglycaemia as a consequence of exercise. Hypoglycaemia may occur some hours after exercise, possibly because the liver and muscles are still replenishing glycogen stores. Exercise may therefore need to be accompanied by extra food, as discussed on p. 25, or by a reduction in insulin dosage, or by a combination of extra food and less insulin. Which approach is used will depend on individual preference, though most patients prefer to take extra food and leave the insulin dose constant. There is considerable individual variation in the amount of extra food or reduction in insulin dosage required. Fingerprick blood sampling before and after exercise can be helpful in insulin treated patients.

TABLE 2 SPORTS WHICH ARE BEST AVOIDED BY INSULIN TREATED PATIENTS

● Mountaineering	● Hang-gliding
● Potholing	● Motor racing
● Deep-sea diving	● Long distance solo yachting

■ Driving

Hypoglycaemia is one of the more common medical causes of road accidents. Patients, even those on a diet, have a statutory responsibility to inform the DVLC of the diagnoses of diabetes and should also inform their insurance companies. The law regards a hypoglycaemic driver as one who is driving under the influence of drugs and it is essential that diabetic drivers know what action to take if they do have a hypo while driving (Table 3).

Ordinary driving licences

The DVLC usually issues licences which are valid for three years at a time subject to a satisfactory medical report. If the DVLC hears of a patient who has had a hypo while driving, the patient's licence is usually withdrawn until the DVLC is satisfied that good diabetic control has been re-established for several months.

Professional driving

Insulin treated patients are not allowed to hold HGV or PSV licences. Patients treated with oral agents must be on short-acting sulphonylureas or biguanides, and the examining doctor must be satisfied that the patient will observe his therapeutic regimen. Taxi drivers are licensed by local councils, and policies vary from one council to another; there are some who will licence insulin treated patients.

TABLE 3 ADVICE TO DRIVERS

Always inform the DVLC
Always inform your insurance company
Always keep glucose tablets in the car

Never drink alcohol and drive
Never drive if you have missed a meal or a snack

If you have a hypo while driving
1. Reach for your glucose tablets and park as quickly and safely as possible
2. Remove the key from ignition, and if alone in the car move into passenger seat
3. Don't start driving until you are sure that the hypo has passed

Assessing fitness to drive

If you are asked to provide a report for the DVLC the major points which need consideration are hypoglycaemia, eyesight, neuropathy and any concomitant illness such as ischaemic heart disease.

Hypoglycaemia

Ask about **frequency** and **severity** of attacks, and also whether warning symptoms are experienced. Frequent hypos are not necessarily a contra-indication to driving if the patient can recognise the onset of an attack and treat it in its early stages. However, patients who get no warning or whose earliest symptom is confusion should not be allowed to drive, even if their attacks are infrequent.

Eyesight

The required standard of visual acuity (clean car number plate at 25 yards in bright sunlight with spectacles if worn) equates to about 6/15 on the Snellen chart. Patients with severe retinopathy and those who have had laser treatment may have visual field defects, or difficulty with light–dark adaptation which could affect night driving. It is usually sufficient to examine visual fields by simple clinical examination; if perimetry is required the DVLC can ask for an ophthalmologist's report.

Neuropathy

Neuropathy is occasionally so severe that the patient is unaware of the position of his feet.

General attitude

You may think it appropriate to state that the patient is compliant with his therapy, attends regularly for supervision and takes a responsible attitude to his diabetes. On some occasions you may think it in everyone's interests to say exactly the opposite!

Medical reports for driving insurance

Some companies ask the doctor to sign a statement to the effect that 'The patient does not represent any additional risk above normal when being considered for motor insurance'. This cannot be so for insulin treated patients in whom there is always a potential risk of hypoglycaemia. In such cases it is best to strike out the offending sentence and replace it with the statement, 'He represents no greater risk than any other patient satisfactorily stabilised on insulin therapy'.

■ Assurance policies and pension schemes

Most companies ask diabetic people for additional premiums for life assurance, for term insurance policies such as those linked to endowment mortgages, and for sickness insurance. For motor insurance some companies will quote the usual rates and others will ask for an additional premium. The best advice for patients is to join the British Diabetic Association which can put them in touch with brokers who have specialist experience of insurance policies for diabetic people. This is often essential for travel insurance because most policies exclude any pre-existing illness.

Pension schemes and superannuation rights should not be affected by diabetes.

■ Foreign travel

Crossing time zones

The commonest enquiry about foreign travel is from an insulin treated patient whose journey will involve crossing time zones. Travelling westward the day is longer (by about 5–8 hours on a transatlantic flight) and travelling eastward the day is shorter. Before giving specific advice ask the patient to obtain the flight departure and arrival times. For example, a patient on twice daily insulin who leaves England at 3.00 p.m. and arrives in New York at 5.00 p.m. local time (but 10.00 p.m. on his biological clock) can take an extra injection of short-acting insulin to cover the in-flight evening meal and then take his usual evening insulin before his second evening meal in New York. When he returns home the day is shorter and if, for example, the flight leaves New York at 8.00 p.m., the evening dose of the longer acting insulin should be reduced by 20–30%.

If in doubt ask your local diabetes clinic for advice.

General advice

Answers to some other questions which patients may ask, or may not think to ask, about foreign travel can be conveniently considered under the following three headings.

1. *Before you go*
   i. *Contact the Airline.* Confirm departure and arrival times and enquire about in-flight meal times. 'Diabetic diets' supplied by some airlines may not contain enough carbohydrate. Specify exactly what you

need, or choose from the standard meal and supplement it with your own extra carbohydrate if necessary.

ii. *Arrange health insurance.* Declare your diabetes. Remember that insurance policies provided as part of a package holiday may exclude pre-existing medical conditions. If travelling to a country with poor health services consider paying the extra premium for air ambulance cover in case you need to return to the UK urgently for treatment. You can get free treatment in EEC countries provided you have obtained the appropriate documents (apply on Form E111 available from your local DHSS office).

iii. *Take your diabetic card.* The British Diabetic Association provides members with a translation of the wording on the card. Make sure the details of your treatment are up to date. Your diabetic card can be very useful if you need treatment or if you have to explain to an immigration officer why you are carrying syringes.

iv. *Obtain supplies* of insulin, syringes, needles, urine/blood test strips, glucose tablets and glucagon. Take more than you need. Do not rely on getting supplies abroad.

v. *Other useful medicines.* Your doctor can advise you what to get. Some medicines may need a private prescription as 'holiday medicines' are not provided by the NHS. Tummy bug pills can be very useful on foreign holidays, and if you are a poor traveller take something for travel sickness. Some anti-vomiting pills can make you drowsy, so try them out at home before you go.

vi. *Vaccination certificates.* Your doctor will advise on what you need. Your requirements are the same as for any non-diabetic traveller.

2. *On the journey*

i. *Carry all essential items in your hand baggage* in case your main luggage goes astray. Some experienced travellers take all their 'diabetic kit' in their hand baggage. Do not put insulin in your main luggage on long flights — it may get frozen in the hold of the aeroplane.

ii. *Allow for long delays at airports*, especially abroad where you may not be able to purchase food. Carry a packet of biscuits in your hand luggage, as well as the glucose which you must always have in your pocket.

iii. *If you have ordered a special diet* remind the cabin staff before you take off.

iv. *If you are travelling alone*, and are on insulin, it is sensible to tell one of the cabin staff in case you have a hypo.

    v. *Altitude enhances the effect of alcohol.* This may confuse any hypo
       (insulin reaction) feelings if you have drunk too much.
  vi. *Sugar-free chewing gum* helps to prevent ears popping on take-off and
       landing.

3. *While abroad*
    i. *Food is often very different.* Test your urine or blood more often.
    ii. *Exercise can cause hypoglycaemia* (insulin reaction). If you are more
       vigorous than usual, e.g. swimming, ski-ing, you will need to eat more
       or reduce your insulin (see p. 25).
  iii. *Sightseeing can put extra strain on your feet.* Wear good quality,
       comfortable shoes, and make sure they are in sound repair.
  iv. *Injecting into sunburnt skin* is no fun.
    v. *Keep insulin out of direct sunlight* and in the coolest place available.
       Cover it with a damp flannel or keep it in a polystyrene box. A fridge
       is not usually necessary.
  vi. *If you need medical advice or treatment.* Seek help sooner than later.
       If possible find an English-speaking doctor. The British Embassy or
       Consul may be able to advise you where best to go for help.

■ Coping with changes in daily routine

Alterations in daily routine can cause significant planning problems for
insulin treated patients.

An evening out with friends may mean that the evening meal is two or
three hours later than usual, e.g. at 8.00 p.m. rather than 6.00 p.m., with a
potential risk of hypoglycaemia between these hours. This can be avoided
by eating the portions which would normally be eaten before bedtime at the
normal evening mealtime and delaying the evening injection of insulin until
shortly before the main meal is eaten at 8.00 p.m. A reminder about the
hypoglycaemic potential of alcohol (Chapter 12) is often appropriate on
these occasions.

After a night out the patient may want to 'lie-in' next morning, but this
can cause hypoglycaemia if breakfast is delayed too long, particularly if the
patient is sufficiently misguided to inject his insulin and then return to bed
without eating. The safest advice is to get up, inject insulin and eat breakfast at the normal time, and then go back to bed.

Shift work can pose problems for insulin treated patients but these are
never insuperable if the patient is prepared to make some extra effort. The
Novopen system or, in some cases, an insulin infusion pump allow con-

siderable changes in daily routine while maintaining good diabetic control if the patient is prepared to monitor his blood glucose regularly.

Mental stress

Severe mental stress can seriously disrupt diabetic control and patients who are going through a divorce or who have suffered a bereavement may experience temporary loss of diabetic control. This may take the form of sustained hyperglycaemia or blood glucose concentrations which fluctuate rapidly between hyper- and hypoglycaemia. The problem may be compounded by the altered eating habits, either anorexia or binge-eating, which can occur with stress. The patient should be encouraged to eat as near normally as possible and to test blood or urine glucoses more frequently. The dose of insulin or oral hypoglycaemic should be adjusted to correct severe hyperglycaemia and minimise hypoglycaemia, but in the short term it is unnecessary to strive for perfect diabetic control which is often unattainable at such times.

Diabetic identity cards

Patients treated with insulin or oral hypoglycaemic drugs should be encouraged to carry a card stating that they have diabetes and giving details of their treatment. Cards may be obtained from the British Diabetic Association and are also provided by several pharmaceutical companies. Some patients prefer to wear an engraved bracelet or the 'Medic-Alert' necklace.

The British Diabetic Association

The British Diabetic Association is a charity which was founded in 1934 to provide advice and help for those with diabetes and to raise money for research. The small annual subscription is an excellent investment for most patients (see Useful addresses, Appendix 5).

11 SEXUAL FUNCTION, CONTRACEPTION AND PREGNANCY

■ Sexual function in men

Impotence occurs in 30–60% of diabetic men, the prevalence increasing with age. The causes are listed in Table 1.

A careful and unhurried history can avoid much unnecessary investigation. Questions about extramarital relationships are a sensitive matter but should be asked. Some men who fail to achieve an erection with their wives will have tried masturbating to see if this produces an erection. If it does the problem is unlikely to be organic. Early morning erections which are present on waking suggest a psychogenic cause, but do not exclude organic pathology. A sudden onset of erectile failure is often of psychogenic origin whereas a history of more gradual failure usually implies an organic cause. The history should also include a review of all drug therapy and enquiry about alcohol consumption. Intercurrent illness, including episodes of poor diabetic control, may cause temporary impotence. Imagined illness, especi-

TABLE 1 CAUSES OF IMPOTENCE

1. Psychogenic
2. Drugs e.g. thiazides, beta-blockers, methyldopa, tricyclics, spironolactone, oestrogens
3. Alcohol
4. Any acute or severe illness
5. Autonomic neuropathy
6. Vascular insufficiency
7. Endocrine — testosterone deficiency
            — hyperprolactinaemia
8. Previous pelvic or genitourinary surgery or trauma
9. Spinal cord injuries

ally a fear of having contracted a sexually transmitted disease, may sometimes result in impotence.

Clinical examination should include an assessment of testicular size and examination of the penis. The peripheral pulses should be examined for evidence of vascular insufficiency and a neurological examination to look for signs of neuropathy is essential. Blood samples should be sent for measurement of testosterone and prolactin levels if no other cause has been found from the history or clinical examination.

Treatment is of the underlying cause where possible. Vascular reconstruction of diseased pelvic vessels is sometimes successful. The insertion of penile implants is helpful in some cases. Other patients may be helped by self injection of papaverine into the penis prior to intercourse; this should only be done when the patient has been taught by someone, usually a urologist, with experience of the technique.

Ejaculatory disorders are probably common in impotent diabetic men. Retrograde ejaculation may occur because the internal bladder sphincter fails to close during ejaculation, possibly as a result of autonomic neuropathy.

Libido and **fertility** are not affected by diabetes.

Sexual function in women

Menstruation may affect glycaemic control. Some women notice an increase in insulin requirement at the start of, or just prior to, each menstrual period, but a few will report that they need less insulin at this time.

Fertility is probably normal, or only slightly subnormal, provided that glycaemic control is reasonable and there is no significant nephropathy.

In contrast to diabetic men, in whom impotence is common, few diabetic women appear to experience problems with **sexual responsiveness** or orgasmic difficulties. However, there has been little research published on these topics, and the frequency of such problems may therefore have been underestimated. Inadequate vaginal lubrication is an occasional complaint. Vaginal candidiasis is more common in diabetic patients; both the patient and her partner should be treated, and poor glycaemic control should be corrected if possible.

Contraception

Pregnancy has major implications for diabetic patients who should be made aware of the need for effective contraception and of the advantages and disadvantages of the different methods.

Hormonal contraception

The oestrogen component of the combined oral contraceptive pill may cause a small increase in insulin requirement, but a more important consideration is the increased risk of vascular disease in those with diabetes and whether it may be aggravated by hormonal contraception. There are no absolute contraindications to the use of the oral contraceptive in diabetic patients, but it is probably wise to encourage consideration of other contraceptive measures in those at greatest risk of vascular disease, e.g.:

- cigarette smokers
- those with hypertension or hyperlipidaemia
- older patients, e.g. over 35 years
- patients with retinopathy, neuropathy or proteinuria

However it is in these groups that pregnancy carries the greatest risks, and in some cases the risks of prescribing an oral contraceptive, if other measures are unacceptable, may be less than the risks of pregnancy. If so, there is a case for considering the progesterone-only pill which may have lesser vascular side effects. The progesterone-only pill may be a slightly less effective contraceptive than the combined pill, possibly because accidental omission of a single dose is more important. However, if the diabetic patient keeps her pills with her insulin kit she is unlikely to forget to take the pill at the time of her evening insulin injection. This is usually the ideal time at which to take the progesterone-only pill, which has its maximum effect about six hours after ingestion.

Intrauterine devices

These may carry a slightly higher risk of intrautrine infection in diabetic patients, but the evidence is not conclusive. There is some evidence that IUDs are slightly less effective in diabetic patients during the first 18 months after insertion.

Mechanical methods

These are safe and effective if properly used, and are often the method of choice, provided that they are acceptable to the patient and her partner.

Sterilisation

This is often preferable to contraception once the family is complete, and provided that the marriage is stable and that the partners are unlikely to separate and remarry. Vasectomy in the non-diabetic man should be con-

sidered in preference to tubal ligation in the diabetic woman, provided that
the woman has a reasonable life expectancy.

■ Pregnancy

Pregnancy has major effects on diabetes, and the diabetic state can influence
the outcome of the pregnancy. The relationships between diabetes and
pregnancy are summarised in Table 2.

Maternal consequences

The renal threshold for glucose (and sometimes also for ketones) decreases
during pregnancy, and pregnant patients must use blood tests rather than

---

TABLE 2 MATERNAL DIABETES AND PREGNANCY

Maternal effects

1. *On the diabetes*
    i. Renal threshold for glucose decreases
    ii. Insulin requirements increase
    iii. Dietary requirements may alter
    iv. Retinopathy and nephropathy may deteriorate

2. *On the pregnancy*
    i. †Pre-eclampsia and toxaemia⎱more common than in
    ii. †Hydramnios   ⎰   non-diabetics

Effects on the fetus

Increased risk of:
1. Spontaneous abortion
2. ★Congenital abnormalities
3. †Macrosomia and late intrauterine death
4. †Respiratory distress syndrome
5. †Hypoglycaemia
6. Hypocalcaemia and hypomagnesaemia
7. Polycythaemia, jaundice

---

†*Minimised by good glycaemic control during pregnancy.*
★*Minimised by good glycaemic control at time of conception and during early
  pregnancy.*

urine tests to monitor their glycaemic control. Insulin requirements increase as a consequence of hormonal changes, and the patient's dietary needs may also need to be reassessed. Diabetic retinopathy and nephropathy may deteriorate and must be monitored carefully. Pre-eclampsia, toxaemia and hydramnios are more common than in non-diabetic patients, but the frequency of these complications can be reduced by ensuring excellent glycaemic control during the pregnancy.

Effects on the fetus

Spontaneous abortion probably occurs more commonly in diabetic women and may be related to the greater prevalence of congenital abnormalities in their offspring. There is evidence that the frequency of congenital abnormalities is related to hyperglycaemia during the early weeks of pregnancy. Maternal hypoglycaemia does not seem to affect teratogenesis. Macrosomia, late intrauterine death, respiratory distress syndrome and neonatal hypoglycaemia are all more common in the babies of diabetic mothers and their frequency can be minimised by avoiding hyperglycaemia during pregnancy.

Prepregnancy counselling

Before the introduction of insulin in 1922 maternal mortality rates were as high as 30% and the fetal and perinatal mortality rate was 30–40%. During the period from 1940–1960 the fetal and perinatal mortality rate was still about 20%, but by the 1970s had fallen to around 5%, and a few centres are now reporting rates as low as 2%. The most common cause of fetal and perinatal morality is now congenital malformation, which occurs about three times more commonly in the children of diabetic mothers compared with children of non-diabetic mothers. There is good evidence that the higher than normal rate of congenital malformations is related to the quality of diabetic control at the time of conception and during the early weeks of pregnancy. It follows that **prepregnancy counselling is essential**.

The aims of prepregnancy counselling are:

1. To explain the reasons for good diabetic control prior to conception and during the pregnancy. Patient motivation is more likely if the reasons are adequately explained.
2. To ensure that diabetic control is as good as possible in any patient who is intending to conceive.

3. To consider contra-indications to pregnancy. Contra-indications as a consequence of diabetes are now rare. Proliferative retinopathy is often made worse by pregnancy but can usually be satisfactorily controlled by laser treatment. However, patients with active retinopathy should consider postponing pregnancy until the retinopathy has been treated. Severe nephropathy or autonomic neuropathy are likely to present major problems during pregnancy and these patients require expert counselling.

4. To give more general advice. For example a woman with diabetes should consider starting a family earlier rather than later in life when the hazards of pregnancy are greater and diabetic complications more likely to have appeared. In addition to the work of bringing up a family she must allow time each day for her own diabetic management, and it is therefore sensible to plan a reasonable interval between each pregnancy and to consider limiting the size of the family to two or three children. Prepregnancy counselling also provides an opportunity to review contraceptive precautions and to advise against smoking and excessive alcohol consumption.

Management during pregnancy and labour

Management during pregnancy and labour should be **supervised by a consultant diabetologist and obstetrician**, although the general practitioner will usually still contribute to the antenatal care. Until recently the usual practice was to admit patients routinely during the later weeks of the pregnancy to ensure good diabetic control and to induce labour at about 36 weeks to minimise the risk of late intrauterine death. The availability of home blood glucose monitoring has meant that hospital admission to ensure good diabetic control is now rarely necessary. With better standards of diabetic control the risk of late intrauterine death is small and probably less than the risks associated with prematurity, so that most diabetologists and obstetricians are now prepared to let the pregnancy continue until after the 38th week or even to term.

During labour the diabetes is usually best managed with an intravenous infusion of insulin and dextrose. Following delivery the insulin dosage decreases rapidly, often returning to prepregnancy levels within 24 hours. On discharge from hospital it is wise to adjust the insulin dosage so that the prandial blood glucose is a little high, about 9 mmol/l, to allow for the extra exercise involved in looking after the new baby. The dose can be adjusted after a few days at home.

Gestational diabetes

Gestational diabetes refers to diabetes which appears during pregnancy and disappears in the puerperium (see Chapter 3). Congenital malformations are no more common in the children of these patients than in the children of non-diabetic mothers, but the other problems associated with diabetic pregnancy listed in Table 2 can still occur. Management is therefore exactly the same as in patients with established diabetes.

Up to 50% of those with gestational diabetes will develop permanent diabetes over the next seven years. They should, therefore, remain under annual review, and should be advised to eat a healthy diet and to keep their weight as near as possible to the ideal for their height and age.

Glucose tolerance tests in pregnancy

The finding of glycosuria is most commonly due to the lowered renal threshold for glucose which occurs during pregnancy but, because of the serious implications of a diagnosis of diabetes, it must always be investigated further.

If any of the risk factors for gestational diabetes (see Chapter 3, Table 2) are present then an oral glucose tolerance test should be arranged. The criteria for a diagnosis of gestational diabetes are given in Chapter 3 (p. 12). If no risk factors are present then measurement of a fasting blood glucose concentration will suffice. A result of less than 5.8 mmol/l in a venous sample may be regarded as normal.

A normal glucose tolerance test in early pregnancy does not preclude the possibility of gestational diabetes occurring later, and if glycosuria persists then a fasting blood glucose or glucose tolerance test should be repeated at about 32 weeks gestation.

Will my baby have diabetes?

This question is often asked by potential or expectant diabetic parents. The answer is that the likelihood of diabetes developing during infancy is extremely small, but there is an increased risk of the child becoming diabetic as time goes by. Nearly all the parents who ask this question will have Type I diabetes, and the diabetic tendency in such cases is closely related to the HLA haplotype, i.e. to the composition of the histocompatibility antigens. As regards the risk of a child developing diabetes it does not therefore matter whether it is the father or the mother who has diabetes. It is not possible to give precise figures but if only one parent is diabetic the risk for each child is between about 1 in 25 and 1 in 80, and if both parents are diabetic the risk is increased to between about 1 in 3 and 1 in 25. If a brother or sister has Type I diabetes then about 1 in 20 siblings will develop diabetes by the age of 16 and about 1 in 13 by the age of 30. More precise figures can be given if HLA typing is carried out.

The risks are much greater in families with non-insulin dependent diabetes, and expert genetic counselling may be required in these cases.

■ Further reading

Burden A.C. (1985). Diabetic control during pregnancy. *Practical Diabetes* 2(5), 16–17.

Ewing D.J. (1985). Sexual dysfunction in diabetic men. *Practical Diabetes* 2(2), 6–9.

Gingell J.C. and Desai K.M. (1987). Investigation of impotence with particular reference to the diabetic. *Practical Diabetes* 4(6), 257–260.

Gorsuch A.N., Gale E.M., Bottazzo G. and Bottazzo F. (1987). Will this child get diabetes? Lessons from family studies. *Treating Diabetes* (Servier Laboratories Ltd) 10, 6–11.

Moley K.H., DeCherney A.H. and Diamond M.P. (1988). Diabetes mellitus in pregnancy: implication in developmental abnormalities. *Practical Diabetes* 5(5), 221–225.

Steel J.M. (1985). Sexual function in diabetic women. *Practical Diabetes* 2(2), 10–11.

Steel J.M. (1985). The pre-pregnancy clinic. *Practical Diabetes* 2(6), 8–10.

12 ALCOHOL AND DIABETES

Our ability to advise patients about alcohol consumption is limited by lack of knowledge about the effects of alcohol on diabetic control and diabetic complications, and some of the advice is necessarily empirical.

■ Some metabolic effects of alcohol

Alcohol is rich in calories (7 kcal per gram). A pint of beer may contain over 100 kcal from alcohol alone and the total energy content will be supplemented by the carbohydrate content which varies considerably in different beers. Those who are overweight should limit their consumption.
Alcohol can cause hypoglycaemia. This may occur in two ways. First, alcohol can inhibit hepatic gluconeogenesis (the synthesis of glucose from non-carbohydrate precursors). Secondly, it can potentiate the effect of insulin which is secreted in response to rapidly absorbed carbohydrate such as sucrose which is consumed with the alcohol.

Less commonly alcohol may cause **hyperglycaemia and ketosis**. The hyperglycaemia can occur because of the high sugar content of some drinks and also because alcohol can inhibit the use of glucose in muscle. Ketosis may occur in malnourished alcoholics who have poor stores of glycogen and are dependent on lipolysis for energy.

Alcohol can cause **hypertriglyceridaemia**. Moderate consumption can increase HDL cholesterol but probably has no effect of total cholesterol concentrations.

■ Diabetic control and diabetic complications

Prolonged, heavy consumption of alcohol can cause glucose intolerance in non-diabetics but the long-term effects of alcohol ingestion on glycaemic control in diabetic patients has not been investigated. The clinical impression that diabetic control is poor in those diabetics who are also alcoholics may reflect poor compliance with treatment rather than a direct effect of alcohol.

There is some evidence that symptomatic peripheral neuropathy and retinopathy are more common in those who take more than 20 drinks per week.

■ Alcohol and oral hypoglycaemic agents

Some pharmacists now label all prescriptions of chlorpropamide with a injunction to 'avoid alcohol', because a minority of patients on this treatment will notice facial flushing when they drink alcohol. All patients for whom chlorpropamide is prescribed should be warned of the possibility of facial flushing, but very few are really bothered by it, and these patients should be offered another medication. The 'avoid alcohol' label sometimes appears on prescriptions of metformin and this is also unjustified. Toxic doses of metformin and alcohol abuse can both cause lactic acidosis, but clinical experience has shown that it is perfectly safe for patients treated with metformin to take small amounts of alcohol, e.g. one or two drinks daily.

Acute ingestion of alcohol can inhibit the metabolism of tolbutamide whereas prolonged heavy consumption increases its metabolism. It is not known if these effects are of clinical importance.

■ Some practical considerations

How much alcohol is safe?

In line with recommendations made by the Royal Colleges of Physicians and Psychiatrists, the British Diabetic Association has suggested that three drinks daily is the maximum safe consumption and that it is better to drink less. Intermittent consumption is safer than regular daily drinking. One drink is defined as half a pint of beer or lager, a single pub measure of spirits (24 cc or $\frac{1}{6}$ gill), or one small glass of wine or sherry. Alcohol should be avoided during pregnancy because of the risk to the fetus which is already greater than normal in the case of diabetic mothers.

Should the calorie and carbohydrate content of the drink be counted in the daily allowance?

Patients who are on a calorie controlled diet **should always count the**

calorie content of any alcoholic drink. Ideally, those patients on a weight reducing diet should abstain from alcohol, but if they must drink they should limit their calorie consumption from alcohol to no more than 10 % of their daily calorie allowance, i.e. a maximum of one drink daily on a 1000 kcal diet.

By contrast the **carbohydrate content of alcoholic drinks should not be counted** in the daily carbohydrate allowance, **provided** that the 'safe maximum' figure of three drinks in any one day is observed. To replace carbohydrate from food with rapidly absorbed sugars in drinks would put the patient at risk of hypoglycaemia some hours later.

Are some drinks preferable to others?

Low carbohydrate beers, lagers and ciders are sometimes promoted as being especially suitable for diabetics, but there is no convincing evidence that this is so, and indeed the reverse may be true. Many such drinks contain more alcohol than do ordinary beers and lagers and this, together with a low carbohydrate content, may increase the risk of hypoglycaemia.

Patients are usually advised to avoid sweet sherries, sweet wines and liqueurs. This advice is entirely empirical. A glass of sweet sherry contains about 6 grams of carbohydrate which is no more than that found in half a pint of many beers. A total embargo on sweet sherries, sweet wines and liqueurs is probably unnecessary.

Hypoglycaemia

Patients must be warned about the potential for alcohol to cause hypoglycaemia. This applies not only to insulin treated patients but also to those given oral hypoglycaemics. Patients need to be aware that **hypoglycaemia can occur several hours after they have finished drinking**. Alcohol is best taken with food, and this food should contain some slowly absorbed (high fibre) carbohydrate to minimise the risk of late hypoglycaemia. Rapidly absorbed carbohydrate is best avoided in those on oral hypoglycaemics because it may increase the chances of a late reactive hypoglycaemia when alcohol is consumed by those patients who can still secrete their own insulin.

◼ Summary of recommendations to patients

The following recommendations are based on those produced by the British Diabetic Association (Connor and Marks, 1985).

1. No more than three drinks in any one day. It is better to drink less, and safer not to drink every day. A drink is defined as $\frac{1}{2}$ pint of beer, lager or cider or single pub measures of spirits ($\frac{1}{6}$ gill), sherry ($\frac{1}{3}$ gill) or wine (4 fl oz).
2. The calorie content of the drink should be counted in the daily calorie allowance by those on calorie controlled diets and should not exceed 10 % of total calorie consumption.
3. The carbohydrate content should **not** be counted in the daily allowance so long as Recommendation 1 is observed. However mixers, such as tonics, cordials, etc., should be of the slimline or low sugar variety.
4. Avoid beers and lagers with a very high or very low carbohydrate content or with a very high alcohol content. Use the information in *Countdown* (1985) to choose a beer with a carbohydrate content of 3–7 grams per half pint and an alcohol concentration of $< 5 \%$ v/v. About half of all beers and lagers sold in the UK meet these criteria.
5. Warn patients that hypoglycaemia may occur several hours after drinking alcohol, and food containing unrefined carbohydrate should always be eaten with, or soon after, drinking. Rapidly absorbed carbohydrate, including that in ordinary tonic waters and cordials, should be avoided to minimise the risk of late reactive hypoglycaemia.
6. Warn patients treated with chlorpropamide about possible facial flushing.

■ Further reading

BDA. *Countdown* (2nd edn). British Diabetic Association, London, 1985.

Connor H. and Marks V. (1985). Alcohol and diabetes. *Diabetic Medicine* 2, 413–416.

Connor H. (1987). Alcohol and diabetes — what should we tell our patients? *Practical Diabetes* 4, 159–160.

Simpson H.C.R. (1987). Metabolic effects of alcohol in diabetes. *Practical Diabetes* 4, 156–158.

13 | DIABETES AND OTHER MEDICAL CONDITIONS

■ Hypertension

Hypertension is commonly present in diabetic patients and is associated with an increased morbidity and mortality. When present, it has an adverse influence on the course of the disease especially if retinopathy or nephropathy coexist. The scale of the problem is staggering: in a large prospective ongoing study of Type II diabetes, about half of the newly-diagnosed diabetic patients were found to be hypertensive.

When to treat hypertension in diabetes

Studies of normal, healthy non-diabetic populations have shown that both systolic and diastolic pressure rise with age. Thus mean blood pressure for a 20 year old may be 120/75 and for a 70 year old 160/85. These facts must be considered before deciding whether or not a patient requires therapy. Moreover, the chances of finding an underlying cause for hypertension decrease with age. For a 50 year old subject the likelihood of an identifiable cause (e.g. renal disease, Cushing's disease) is less than 10%; for a 70 year old it is less than 5%. The decision as to whether or not treatment is required therefore depends on age and also the presence or absence of long-term complications such as retinopathy or nephropathy. In the latter case, aggressive anti-hypertensive therapy can preserve renal function and should therefore be attempted. Guidelines for treatment of hypertension in diabetic subjects without proliferative retinopathy or nephropathy are given in Table 1.

Every diabetic patient should have his blood pressure checked at least annually and, if found to be hypertensive, the subsequent course of action depends on other findings at the annual review. If the analysis reveals

TABLE 1 DEFINITIONS OF HYPERTENSION (Suggested criteria for treatment of 'essential' hypertension in uncomplicated diabetes)

		Systolic	Diastolic
WHO definition {	Normotension	< 140	< 90
	Hypertension	< 160	> 95
When to treat?			
Diabetes, age under 60		> 150	> 95
Diabetes, age over 60		> 160	> 100

proteinuria in a 50 year old, Type I diabetic patient with treated retinopathy and a BP of 160/100, then further investigations are indicated and may be best arranged by the hospital diabetic clinic. These would normally include a full screening of serum biochemistry, a 24 hour urine collection for creatinine clearance and protein excretion, chest X-ray and ECG. However, a 50 year old obese Type II diabetic patient with the same BP but no proteinuria or other complications would not require such intensive investigation. An approach to such a patient is provided in the following section.

How to manage the hypertensive patient

1. *Is the diagnosis confirmed?*
   - Hypertension should generally only be diagnosed if three readings on separate occasions meet the criteria shown in Table 1. However, there are exceptions to this rule, e.g. a patient with clinical, electrocardiographical and radiological evidence of cardiomegaly, together with diabetic retinopathy would require immediate treatment if found to have a significantly elevated blood pressure.
   - A large cuff should be used in the very obese patient.

2. *Is there an identifiable cause?*
   - A history of renal disease should be sought.
   - Is dipstick-positive proteinuria present? If confirmed on two samples in a hypertensive diabetic patient, consider hospital referral for investigation.

3. *Is another medication contributing?*
   - Other prescribed medications (e.g. contraceptive pill, antacids with high salt content, non-steroidal anti-inflammatory drugs) may be exacerbating the problem.

4. *Consider non-pharmacological advice first*
   - *Weight* — the obese patient may simply require reinforcement of a high fibre, low fat diet.
   - *Salt intake* — reduction of sodium intake may be beneficial. Advise a 'no added' salt diet and reduce high salt food consumption (e.g. potato crisps, savoury snacks).
   - *Alcohol* — a high alcohol intake may contribute to a raised blood pressure. Reduction of alcohol consumption may be beneficial.

5. *If BP remains high, consider drug therapy*
   The commonly used drugs are listed in Table 2. Many antihypertensive agents can adversely affect glucose tolerance and serum lipid concentrations and therefore the merits and disadvantages of each class of drug will be considered.
   i. *Beta-blocking drugs.* These are commonly prescribed first-line anti-hypertensive medication in essential hypertension. Although beta-blockers can impair the insulin response to glucose, mask some hypoglycaemic symptoms and adversely affect lipids, use of cardio-selective agents such as Atenolol or Metoprolol may be associated with fewer such problems. If caution is exercised in insulin treated patients, beta-blockers can be extremely effective in managing mild to moderate hypertension in diabetic patients. **Remember** — do not use if cardiac failure, peripheral vascular disease (both of which are more common in diabetic patients) or asthma are present.

   ii. *Calcium channel blockers.* These are useful in the first line management of hypertension in diabetic patients. The occasional unpleasant side effects (facial flushing, light-headedness) may be reduced by starting with a relatively low dose (e.g. Nifedipine Retard 10 mg b.d.) and increasing as necessary.

   iii. *Angiotensin converting enzyme (ACE) inhibitors.* This relatively new class of antihypertensive agent is being increasingly used in the management of hypertension in diabetes with good effect. There do not appear to be any adverse effects of ACE inhibitors on glucose control or lipids, and when used with a thiazide, the adverse effects

TABLE 2 ANTIHYPERTENSIVE THERAPY FOR DIABETIC PATIENTS

Class	Proper name	Trade name	Dosage (mg)		Notes
Beta-blockers	Atenolol	Tenormin	50–100	**Avoid:**	in asthma, peripheral vascular disease, cardiac failure
	Metoprolol	Betaloc	100–400		
		Lopressor		**Caution:**	in insulin treated patients
Calcium channel blockers	Nifedipine	Adalat Retard	10–40	Gradual increase of dose to minimise side effects	
	Nicardipine	Cardene	60–120		
	Verapamil	(Multiple)	40–320		
ACE inhibitors	Captopril	Capoten Acepril	6.25–100	**Caution:**	if renal impairment, start with low dose and gradually increase. Often used with diuretic
	Enalopril	Innovace	2.5–40		

Thiazide diuretics	Bendrofluazide (example)		2.5–10	**Caution:** may worsen diabetic control, cause hypokalaemia, and worsen hyperlipidaemia
Other agents	Hydralazine	Apresoline	25–200	Vasodilators: side effects not uncommon; not first-line agents
	Prazosin	Hypovase	0.5–20	
	Indapamide	Natrilix	2.5	Vasorelaxant: do not use with thiazide diuretics
	Methyldopa	Aldomet	125–3000	Centrally acting drug

Note: This table is not comprehensive but provides examples of the more commonly used drugs.

of the latter drug may be reduced. A low initial dose with gradual increases reduces the chance of side effects developing. Hyperkalaemia may develop in patients with renal impairment and electrolytes should be monitored.

iv. *Thiazide diuretics*. Although the thiazides are an alternative first-line treatment for essential hypertension in the non-diabetic population, their adverse effects on glycaemia and lipids are such that they **should not be a first choice in diabetic patients**. However, the diabetogenic effect of the thiazide diuretics is reversible and, as stated above, they may be used with ACE inhibitors with good effect.

v. *Other antihypertensive agents*. A number of other anti-hypertensive agents are also commonly used and a list is given in Table 2.

Summary

The approach to hypertension in diabetes should be as follows:

1. **Confirm diagnosis** — at least three elevated readings unless the pressure is very high or there is evidence of hypertensive end-organ damage.
2. Consider possible treatable causes.
3. Try non-pharmacological intervention.
4. If BP still elevated, consider beta-blocker, calcium channel blocker or ACE inhibitor as drug of first choice.

Note: Patients with diabetic nephropathy require a more aggressive approach to treatment (see Chapter 8).

Hyperlipidaemia

Hyperlipidaemia contributes to the increased risk of vascular disease in diabetic patients.

Causes of hyperlipidaemia in diabetic patients

1. *Poor diabetic control*
   The effects of poor diabetic control on serum lipid concentrations are summarised in Table 3. **Raised** concentrations of LDL cholesterol

TABLE 3 GLYCAEMIC CONTROL AND LIPOPROTEIN CONCENTRATIONS

Lipoprotein	Associated lipid	Glycaemic control	
		Poor	Good
VLDL	Mainly triglyceride	↑↑	N
LDL	Mainly cholesterol	↑/N	N
HDL	Mainly cholesterol	↓	N

(cholesterol which is associated with low-density lipoprotein) and of triglyceride, and **low** concentrations of HDL cholesterol (cholesterol which is associated with high-density lipoprotein) may all contribute to the risk of vascular disease. It is evident from Table 3 that results of lipid analyses in diabetic patients must be interpreted in the light of other measures of diabetic control, such as blood glucose and glycosylated haemoglobin concentrations.

2. *Obesity*
Obesity is common in NIDDM and is often associated with increased concentrations of VLD (very low density) lipoprotein. Serum triglyceride concentrations may be increased and there may be a modest increase in cholesterol concentrations. These effects are corrected by weight loss.

3. *Diabetic nephropathy*
This is associated with hypercholesterolaemia.

4. *Familial hyperlipidaemia*
Familial hypertriglyceridaemia may be associated with obesity and resistance to the action of insulin. Other types of hyperlipidaemia are not genetically co-inherited with diabetes although the two conditions often co-exist, possibly because of independent associations with other metabolic problems such as obesity.

5. *Other causes of hyperlipidaemia (Table 4)*
Alcohol can cause hypertriglyceridaemia. In some patients this occurs with quite modest alcohol consumption, and a trial of abstention from

TABLE 4 OTHER CAUSES OF SECONDARY HYPERLIPIDAEMIA

- Alcohol
- Drugs
  —oestrogens, including combined oral contraceptive
  —beta-blockers
  —thiazides
- Hypothyroidism
- Nephrotic syndrome
- Renal failure
- Cholestasis
- Pregnancy

alcohol can sometimes be justified. Some drugs can impair both gly-caemic and lipid homeostasis, and existing drug therapy should be reviewed. Hypothyroidism can also be associated with hypercholes-terolaemia.

The aims of treatment

The risk of coronary artery disease is approximately doubled as the total serum cholesterol rises from 5 mmol/l to 6.5 mmol/l. Above 6.5 mmol/l the risk increases more steeply. The British Hyperlipidaemia Association (Shepherd *et al.*, 1987) and other organisations have therefore recommen-ded that the aim of treatment should be to achieve a total serum cholesterol concentration as near as possible to 5 mmol/l or less. **A total cholesterol concentration of 5 mmol/l or less should be regarded as the ideal, but not necessarily as a goal which must be achieved in all cases**. Other factors will influence the doctor's decision on how vigorous the treatment should be in the individual patient. Cholesterol concentrations rise with increasing age and one might accept a cholesterol concentration of 6.0 mmol/l in a 50 year old more readily than a 30 year old, but if the 50 year old had a strong family history of coronary artery disease this might influence both the doctor (and patient) to pursue treatment more energeti-cally. When the total cholesterol concentration is only slightly increased, e.g. 6.0–7.0 mmol/l, it may be helpful to measure the **HDL cholesterol**. A raised HDL cholesterol concentration will identify the few patients whose hypercholesterolaemia is due to hyper-alpha-lipoproteinaemia which is a benign condition. In these patients one should aim for an LDL cholesterol (calculated as the total cholesterol minus the HDL cholesterol) of less than 3.5 mmol/l.

The role of **hypertriglyceridaemia** in the causation of vascular disease remains uncertain and criteria for treatment are arbitrary. Fasting serum triglyceride concentrations of 3–6 mmol/l are commonly due to obesity or excessive alcohol intake. Concentrations of greater than 6 mmol/l predispose to pancreatitis and should be treated.

Establishing the diagnosis

When to sample?

It is best to wait for two months following the diagnosis of diabetes or after any period of poor diabetic control (See Table 3). Any acute illness can disturb lipid homeostasis, usually depressing cholesterol and raising triglyceride concentrations, and again sampling should be deferred for two months. The first few weeks after Christmas and the New Year may also produce results which are unrepresentative!

Fasting or random samples?

Ideally the sample should be taken after a 14 hour fast because triglyceride concentrations are greatly influenced by food. However this can cause organisational problems, especially for those on insulin. **A reasonable compromise is to take a random sample for total cholesterol concentration**. If the total cholesterol concentration exceeds 6.5 mmol/l, or if the serum is turbid or milky (indicating marked hypertriglyceridaemia) the patient should be recalled for a fasting sample for analysis of total cholesterol and triglyceride concentrations, HDL cholesterol and measurement of lipoprotein concentrations. Interpretation is simplified if samples are also taken for blood glucose and glycosylated haemoglobin concentrations as a measure of glycaemic control.

Subsequent management

Consider the possibility of a secondary hyperlipidaemia (see Table 4), and treat the cause if possible.

Dietary management

The dietary principles outlined for treatment of hyperglycaemia (p. 19–20) will also be sufficient for most of the milder cases of hyperlipidaemia (cholesterol < 6.5 mmol/l and triglycerides < 6.0 mmol/l), although additional cholesterol restriction may be needed in some patients with hypercholesterolaemia. As with diabetes itself, dietary management is the foundation stone of treatment for hyperlipidaemia and success is enhanced by enlisting the help of a dietitian.

A common mistake is to prescribe a low cholesterol diet for patients with hypertriglyceridaemia. The important dietary principles of the treatment of hypertriglyceridaemia are the correction of obesity where applicable and restriction of alcohol consumption. Patients with a fasting triglyceride concentration of > 6 mmol/l should avoid alcohol altogether because of the risk of pancreatitis. Some patients with familial hypertriglyceridaemia associated with markedly increased levels of chylomicrons need very severe fat restriction and substitution of normal dietary fat with medium chain triglycerides; such patients need referral to a specialist physician.

Drug treatment
Drug treatment, **in addition to diet**, is needed for those patients who do not respond to diet alone. Most lipid-lowering drugs are expensive.

Anion exchange resins (Cholestyramine, Colestipol) are used for hypercholesterolaemia, because they bind bile acids in the gut, thereby lowering LDL cholesterol. They sometimes increase VLD lipoprotein concentrations and can therefore aggravate hypertriglyceridaemia, in which case a fibric acid drug may be needed as well as, or in place of, the resin. Gastrointestinal side effects and poor palatibility may limit their acceptability and the dose should be built up gradually to minimise these effects. Anion exchange resins may delay or reduce the absorption of some drugs, e.g. digoxin, warfarin, paracetamol and thyroxin.

Fibric acid drugs (Clofibrate, Bezafibrate, Gemfibrozil). These drugs mainly **decrease triglyceride** concentrations and also increase HDL cholesterol. The effect on LDL cholesterol is variable; it usually decreases but occasionally increases as more VLDL is converted to LDL. Gemfibrozil is the most potent (and most expensive), but bezafibrate, when prescribed as Bezalip-mono, has the advantage of a once daily dosage; both are probably less likely to cause gallstones than is clofibrate. They may cause myositis, especially if renal function is impaired, and can potentiate the effects of oral hypoglycaemics and oral anticoagulants.

Nicotinic acid and **nicofluranose** lower both cholesterol and triglyceride concentrations but cause unpleasant flushing and headaches; they are usually reserved for patients with severe familial hypercholesterolaemia.

Probucol lowers total cholesterol concentrations, but is less often used because it lowers HDL cholesterol as well as LDL cholesterol. **Maxepa** is a concentrated fish oil preparation which lowers VLDL triglyceride and may have beneficial effects on platelet function. Its long-term safety is unproven. The HMG-CoA reductase inhibitor, **Simvastatin**, is now prescribable for patients with primary hypercholesterolaemia, intolerant or unresponsive to other therapies and with a cholesterol > 7.8 mmol/l.

The patient who relapses

Having achieved satisfactory blood lipid concentrations it is essential that the tests be checked at the annual diabetic review. If the results deteriorate the following points should be considered:

Has the diet altered?
An increase in weight or a deterioration in glycaemic control, or a change in social circumstances such as bereavement or leaving home for university may provide clues suggesting a change in eating habits. If in doubt a reassessment by a dietitian may be useful.

Has some secondary cause for hyperlipidaemia supervened?
See Table 4 for secondary causes.

Who should be referred?

Most patients with hyperlipidaemia can be managed by their general practitioners with help from a dietitian but some merit referral to a physician with a specialist interest. The usual indications for referral are outlined below.

Failure to achieve satisfactory results
Referral can be helpful even in those cases where lack of therapeutic success is attributable to poor compliance with diet or drug therapy. A second opinion may sometimes convince the patient of the error of his ways.

Patients with very high lipid concentrations
For example: cholesterol > 10 mmol/l or fasting triglycerides > 10 mmol/l, at the outset are likely to need specialist advice if they are to achieve acceptable results. The specialist may not actually need to see the patient if the referral letter contains all the necessary information, i.e.

1. current blood test results, and the results before any treatment was started;
2. what dietary advice has been given;
3. a list of **all** drug treatment (not just the lipid-lowering agents);
4. the patient's weight and height;
5. any information which may be relevant to possible secondary causes for hyperlipidaemia.

Screening of relatives

In cases of familial hyperlipidaemia the patient should be advised that it would be sensible for his children and siblings to be screened.

■ Intercurrent illness, drug therapy and diabetes

People with diabetes get other illnesses, just like everybody else, but the usual management of the other condition may need to be modified or altered because of the diabetes and, more commonly, the management of the diabetes may need adjustment as a result of the other illness.

Principles of diabetic management during intercurrent illness

Intercurrent illness is usually associated with **resistance to the action of insulin**, and therefore with hyperglycaemia. Diabetic ketoacidosis constitutes a greater risk to the patient's well-being than does the risk of hypoglycaemia which may result from any associated anorexia or vomiting.

All patients (and their doctors) must know:
1. NEVER STOP INSULIN
2. TEST BLOOD/URINE GLUCOSE FREQUENTLY, increase the dose of insulin or oral hypoglycaemic if the tests are high, and seek medical help promptly if hyperglycaemia persists or if there is more than a trace of ketonuria.

The indications for hospital admission are discussed in Chapter 7.

The vomiting diabetic patient

Vomiting may be due to the intercurrent illness, e.g. gastroenteritis or other abdominal pathology, but may also be a symptom of diabetic ketoacidosis. It complicates the diabetic management because of the risk of hypoglycaemia which is mostly likely in insulin treated patients but may also occur in those treated with sulphonylureas.

Even if the patient is nauseated he may still be able to take drinks which contain carbohydrate (see Appendix 2). If vomiting occurs an injection or a suppository of an antiemetic is worth trying, but **if the vomiting persists immediate hospital admission is necessary**.

Acute myocardial infarction

Myocardial infarction occurs twice as commonly in diabetic patients and carries a mortality which is twice as high as in non-diabetic patients.

Acute myocardial infarction is often accompanied by hyperglycaemia. There is some evidence to suggest that the excess mortality may be decreased by use of an intravenous insulin infusion to obtain really good glycaemic control during the first few days after the infarct. **Admission to hospital should always be considered.**

Metformin should be discontinued because heart failure or hypotension will cause hypoxia with a consequent risk of lactic acidosis.

Illness affecting metabolism of oral hypoglycaemic drugs

Illnesses which affect hepatic or renal function may cause accumulation of oral hypoglycaemic drugs, and lead to hypoglycaemia and other toxic side effects. Renal function may be impaired because of non-renal disease, e.g. dehydration or hypotension. Metformin therapy should always be discontinued in patients with renal or hepatic disease because of the risk of lactic acidosis (see Chapter 5).

Drugs which may affect glycaemic control

A list of drugs which affect glycaemic control is given in Appendix 3, and some of those with major effects are discussed below.

Glucocorticoids
The effect is dose-related and is unlikely at doses of less than 7.5 mg daily of prednisolone or its equivalent dose of other steroids. Large doses of inhaled or topically applied steroids may cause glucose intolerance.

Oral contraceptives
Oestrogens only cause glucose intolerance in doses greater than 75 μg daily and the effect of modern oral contraceptives is dependent on the progesterone component. Norethisterone appears to have little or no effect but levonorgestrel in doses of 30 μg or more daily can cause glucose intolerance.

Thiazides and chlorthalidone
These can cause glucose intolerance in normal subjects, but the effect in patients with Type II diabetes is more rapid and more profound, and is accentuated by concurrent therapy with propranolol.

Salbutamol
Salbutamol can cause hyperglycaemia, and when it is used in combination with dexamethasone for pre-term labour the hyperglycaemia can be considerable.

Alcohol
Alcohol can cause hypoglycaemia and can modify the symptoms of hypoglycaemia (see Chapter 12).

Drug interactions
Interactions with sulphonylureas usually result in potentiation of the hypoglycaemic effect, but rifampicin can cause increased metabolism of sulphonylureas leading to hyperglycaemia.

Linctuses
These often contain sugar to make them more palatable. The amounts of glucose are usually small but, when possible, it is better to use a preparation which does not contain sugar. Some sugar-free cough linctuses are listed in Table 5.

Drugs which interfere with urine and blood tests

There are some drugs which may appear to affect diabetic control by causing false-positive or false-negative results with reagent strips. The greatest problems occur with 'Clinitest' tablets which measure reducing substances and are not specific for glucose. False-positive results may occur

TABLE 5 SOME SUGAR-FREE COUGH LINCTUSES

Trade name	Active ingredient	
Galcodine	Codeine	15 mg/5 ml
Galenphol	Pholcodine	5 mg/5 ml
Galenphol strong	Pholcodine	10 mg/5 ml
Diatuss	Pholcodine	10 mg/5 ml
Pavacol-D	Pholcodine	5 mg/5 ml
Pholcomed-D	Pholcodine	5 mg/5 ml
	Papaverine	1.25 mg/5 ml

in patients treated with vitamin C, aspirin, nalidixic acid, cephalosporins, methyldopa, probenecid and some anti-tuberculous drugs.

Reagent strips which use glucose oxidase to measure urine glucose are less susceptible to interference by drugs. However, false-negative results may occur in patients who take large doses of vitamin C and also in those treated with L-dopa. Cephalosporins can produce a black colour with 'Diastix'. Ketonuria may cause a false-negative result with 'Clinistix' but does not significantly affect the result if 'Diastix' or 'Diabur' is used. false-positive results may occur if the urine is passed into a container which has been rinsed in oxidising disinfectants.

Reagent strips for ketones may give false-positive results with L-dopa.

Reagent strips for blood glucose estimation may give falsely low results in patients taking large quantities of vitamin C. The use of an alcohol-containing swab to sterilise the skin before taking the blood sample may also give a falsely low result because alcohol inhibits glucose oxidase.

Further reading

Hypertension

Ritchie C.M. and Atkinson A.B. (1986). Towards better management of the diabetic patient with raised blood pressure. *Diabetic Medicine* **3**, 301–305.

Hyperlipidaemia

Shepherd J., Betteridge D.J., Durrington P., *et al.* (1987). Strategies for reducing coronary heart disease and desirable limits for blood lipid concentrations: guidelines of the British Hyperlipidaemia Association. *British Medical Journal* **295**, 1245–1246.

Intercurrent illness and drug therapy

Drug interactions in diabetics. *Drug and Therapeutic Bulletin*, 1979 **17**, 37–40.

Drugs and glucose tolerance. *Adverse Drug Reaction Bulletin*, 1986 **121**, 452–455.

14 SPECIAL GROUPS

Fortunately, diabetes is relatively rare in childhood and adolescence, with a prevalence of 1–2 per 1000, whereas in the very elderly, the prevalence may be as high as 8%. Some of the problems that are peculiar to the young and the old patient will be discussed in this chapter.

■ Diabetes in children

A recent survey of diabetic control demonstrated the problems of management of young diabetic patients. This group had poor control with less than 2% of patients having glycosylated haemoglobin levels in the normal range.

Presentation

Young children invariably have Type I diabetes and the clinical presentation is usually acute. The patient normally has a short history of classical hyperglycaemic symptoms and may be very ill when medical advice is first sought. The presence of glycosuria is highly significant, and ketonuria should also be sought. An urgent blood glucose test is indicated with immediate hospital referral which should usually be by telephone. A child is more likely than an adult to have ketoacidosis when first diagnosed, and may present as an acute abdominal problem with pain and vomiting. Very young children, in particular, may present diagnostic problems because they may rapidly become dehydrated and tachypnoeic, and be misdiagnosed as having a chest problem. Diabetes should be considered in any child with an acute unexplained illness. Whereas acidotic or dehydrated children always require admission, the policy for the less acutely ill, newly-diagnosed child varies between hospitals, with some promoting initial stabilisation and management at home.

Management

The principles of management are similar to those for the older patient with Type I diabetes, with appropriate dietary advice (see Chapter 4), insulin therapy (Chapter 5), and home blood monitoring. As life expectancy is long, the need to aim for good metabolic control is even more important in the young patient. Children should usually be started on two injections daily, and a soluble and isophane mixture is popular: the multiple injection regimens using devices such as the 'Novopen' are also gaining popularity amongst younger patients.

The diagnosis of diabetes in a child has a profound effect on the whole family, with denial of the diabetes being a common problem in the patient whilst feelings of anxiety and guilt may be experienced by the parents. Careful explanation to the family and emotional support during the first few weeks will help enormously, and the dramatic response of the child to insulin will usually reinforce the optimistic prognosis that can be offered. However, continued support will be needed as the child may soon feel isolated from friends as, for example, common snacks such as chocolate, sweets and crisps are denied or limited to small quantities. Groups and associations such as the British Diabetic Association are able to offer help and advice to families, and many children benefit from attending holidays such as camps and outward-bound courses which are specifically designed to help them cope with diabetes.

Parents will often seek advice on the problems that the child may face at school, especially with reference to sports. Exercise should be encouraged, and with advice on increasing the carbohydrate or reducing the insulin, most school sports are possible for diabetic children. The school pack designed by the British Diabetic Association is particularly helpful for the newly-diagnosed patient going back to school on insulin.

Complications

Although chronic complications are rare, acute problems (see also Chapter 7) are common and both the patient and the family should be able to recognise and manage hypo- and hyperglycaemic emergencies. Hypoglycaemia is the most feared problem amongst young patients and a recent survey suggested that reactions occur at least weekly in most children. Symptoms may be different from, and more variable than those in adults, with facial pallor and altered behaviour being common early signs, whereas sweating tends to be a later manifestation. Early recognition, with confirmation of the diagnosis and appropriate treatment, should form part of the initial education of the patient and the family: this should include the use of glucagon by the parents. After recovery the child should be encouraged to eat or drink the equivalent of 10–20 gram carbohydrate snack.

Hyperglycaemic emergencies may develop with alarming rapidity in children, and **parents should know that insulin should NEVER be stopped,** even when the child is ill and anorexic. The significance of ketonuria and vomiting should also be explained and parents should be encouraged to seek help early during any hyperglycaemic episode. Whereas sick ketoacidotic children should be admitted to hospital, many mild episodes of ketonuria and hyperglycaemia are often easily treated at home and reverse rapidly. Regular monitoring of both blood glucose and ketonuria is required during any acute episodes.

Long-term care

During the first few months after diagnosis, the parents invariably have many questions which may be addressed to the family doctor whom they know, rather than to members of the unfamiliar diabetes team in the Paediatric Outpatient Department. A close relationship is usually formed with the diabetes specialist nurse. These questions commonly include the recognition of, and risks of developing, short- and long-term complications, dietary management at home and school, and alterations of insulin dosage according to results of home blood glucose monitoring. The British Diabetic Association provides much helpful literature for the families of newly-diagnosed diabetic children.

■ Diabetes in adolescence

The turmoil that often accompanies the physical and psychological changes of adolescence may be accentuated in the diabetic patient. Rebellion against the restraints that are imposed by having diabetes is common, and denial that metabolic control is of importance frequently occurs. In addition, hormonal changes may exacerbate the problems and increase the difficulties of achieving good control. Thus the management of the adolescent patient poses both medical and social problems. Co-operation and good communication between hospital and community staff are therefore especially important in this age group. Some hospital diabetes clinic staff have responded by establishing special adolescent clinics, where the specialist nurses and doctors may help to manage and discuss some of the problems that may occur. Confrontation should be avoided and with skill most patients can be guided through these difficult years. Several centres have also responded by forming self-help groups, where patients meet regularly and discuss the problems they face, often with the help of a specialist nurse. Continuing parental support is essential.

Particular problems that may occur include erratic control with frequent hypoglycaemic reactions and excessive weight gain. The aim of education should be to demonstrate to patients that they are in control of their diabetes, and that by monitoring and altering insulin doses as indicated, acute problems may be avoided. The use of too many additional carbohydrate snacks to avoid hypos should be avoided as this can lead to weight gain.

The possibility of anorexia or bulimia nervosa occurring in this age group should be borne in mind. The introduction of pen injection devices, such as the Novopen, has proved popular amongst adolescent patients as it has permitted some increased flexibility of lifestyle which may be accompanied by a reduction in the frequency of hypoglycaemic reactions.

Adolescent girls need advice about contraception and prepregnancy counselling (Chapter 11) and all adolescents should be told about the effects of alcohol on diabetic control (Chapter 12).

The family doctor is an important member of the diabetes team during childhood and adolescence: the patients may move from the paediatric clinic through the adolescent to the adult clinic whereas the GP remains the same. Knowledge of the patients and their family background often helps in their management through adolescence. True brittle diabetes, where life is continually disrupted by recurring hypoglycaemic or hyperglycaemic episodes, is rare and most patients overcome the traditional problems that diabetes poses during puberty and thereafter.

◼ Diabetes in the very elderly

Prevalence

The prevalence of diabetes increases with age so that 4.5% of men and 2.9% of women aged 75 and over will have diabetes (Table 1). The very elderly present special problems of management, partly because of their age and partly because of the frequency of social and other medical problems.

Aims of treatment

It used to be taught that there was less need for good glycaemic control in the elderly because the likelihood of a 75 year old living long enough to develop complications was small. However, many patients with Type II

TABLE 1 THE PREVALENCE OF DIABETES IN THE ELDERLY

Age (years)	Prevalence (% of total population)
All ages	1.0
65–74 male	3.3
female	2.5
75 + male	4.6
female	2.9

Note: Data from Petri et al., 1986.

diabetes will already have complications at the time of diagnosis and these complications may progress more rapidly if glycaemic control is poor. In practice, every patient must be assessed individually. The risks of poor or moderate glycaemic control must be weighed against the potential benefits of good control and the dangers which may be entailed in achieving it. In many cases the balance will be in favour of less intensive management, but this is not invariably so. Much will depend on an assessment of the patient's physical and mental capabilities and on the social circumstances. The information required for such an assessment will usually be known to the family doctor or to other members of the primary health care team, but occasionally a formal assessment of 'daily living' capabilities can be helpful.

Dietary advice

Dietary advice for the very elderly should be explained as simply as possible, and there should be as little interference with the patient's eating habits as is compatible with safe and reasonable diabetic control. It is not usually necessary to insist that an 80 year old should change the habits of a lifetime and eat 30 grams of fibre daily when he or she has been used to only half that amount, and it is certainly not reasonable to restrict cholesterol intake at this stage. Dietary explanation may be needed not only for the patient but also for cooks in old peoples' homes, and special arrangements may have to be made for those who attend luncheon clubs or receive meals-on-wheels.

Treatment with oral hypoglycaemics and insulins

Particular care is required to avoid drug toxicity in the elderly. Drugs which are excreted by the kidneys should be used with special caution because renal function deteriorates with age (see Chapter 5). The frequency of drug treatment for other medical conditions in the elderly increases the potential for drug interactions with oral hypoglycaemic agents.

There is an understandable tendency to postpone insulin therapy for as long as possible in the very elderly, but treatment with insulin should not be withheld if it is justified by the patient's symptoms. Most elderly patients prefer a daily injection to the polyuria which may result in them being labelled as incontinent. It is sometimes assumed that elderly patients will not be capable of giving their own injections. The assumption may be made on the basis of inability to cope with injections while an inpatient in hospital. However, there are some elderly patients who have failed to cope with learning to inject while in hospital but who manage perfectly well when taught in the more comfortable and familiar surroundings of their own home. An elderly patient may not learn the technique as quickly as a younger patient, and patience and understanding are essential. Experimentation with different syringes or with cartridge systems such as the 'Novopen' may be needed to find the best method for the individual. For example, some people with arthritic hands may find that a thicker, glass syringe is easier to hold than a thin, plastic one. Some visually handicapped patients may need a magnifying glass which clips onto the syringe or one of the special types of syringe described in Chapter 5. The advice and experience of a nurse with specialist training in diabetes can be invaluable in these circumstances.

Complications

Avoidance of hypoglycaemia can be of even greater importance in the elderly than in younger patients. Many elderly people live alone and this increases the potential hazards of hypoglycaemia. Hypoglycaemia due to oral hypoglycaemic agents is often of insidious onset with predominantly neuroglycopenic symptoms which may be attributed to confusion from other causes. Hypoglycaemia may predispose to falls and to hypothermia.

Chronic complications are probably commoner in the elderly. In patients aged 65 and over, Petri *et al.* (1986) found evidence of cardiovascular disease in 96% and of retinopathy in 46%, whereas the prevalence of diabetic retinopathy in all diabetic patients is only 20–25%. Diabetic foot problems are commoner and often more disabling in elderly patients. The elderly are more likely to need chiropody. A comprehensive annual review and reinforcement of educational advice are therefore as important in the elderly patients as they are in younger people. It may take longer to examine an elderly and disabled patient and adequate time must be allowed.

▮ Further reading

Diabetes in children

McFarlane P.I. and Smith C.S. (1988). Perceptions on hypoglycaemia in childhood diabetes mellitus: a questionnaire study. *Practical Diabetes* **5**, 56–58.

Kinmonth A.L. (1987). Management of diabetes in childhood. *Prescribers' Journal* **27**, 1–12.

Seminar on Adolescent Diabetes Mellitus. *Practical Diabetes*, 1985, **2**, 20.

Diabetes in the elderly

Arora B.A. and Arora A. (1986). Dietary management in the elderly diabetic. *Practical Diabetes* **3**, 116–118.

Bates A. (1986). Diabetes in old age. *Practical Diabetes* **3**, 120–123.

Caird F.I. (1986). Geriatricians and diabetes. *Practical Diabetes* **3**, 124–125. ·

Petri M.P., Gatling W., Petri L. and Hill R.D. (1986). Diabetes in the elderly — an epidemiological perspective. *Practical Diabetes* **3**, 153–155.

15 THE POORLY-CONTROLLED DIABETIC PATIENT

The management of hypoglycaemia and severe hyperglycaemia has been discussed in Chapter 7. In this chapter the problems of unstable diabetes and moderate, sustained hyperglycaemia will be considered.

Unstable diabetes

The term 'unstable diabetes' is used when the blood glucose concentration fluctuates, often unpredictably and for no immediately obvious reason, between high and low levels. In its most extreme form it constitutes 'brittle diabetes' which is described in more detail below.

The common causes of unstable diabetes are:

1. **Emotional stress** which tends to cause hyperglycaemia but which may also be associated with hypoglycaemia if the emotional upset also causes anorexia or disordered eating patterns. Major fluctuations in blood glucose concentration should also alert the clinician to the possibility of anorexia or bulimia nervosa.
2. **Other organic disease** usually leads to sustained hyperglycaemia, but sometimes causes fluctuation in blood glucose concentrations.
3. **Incorrect insulin type or dosage**: an inadvertent change in the type of insulin, e.g. from a beef to a human isophane or vice versa, may upset diabetic control (see Chapter 5). Patients do not always question the change in insulin which has been dispensed, especially if the labels on the new and the old bottles state that they are both isophane insulins. Now that only 100 strength insulin (100 units per ml) is available in the United Kingdom there is no possibility for confusion between insulin preparations of different strengths, but confusion in dosage can still occur with changes in syringes. On the 1 ml syringe each graduation represents 2 units, but on the 0.5 ml syringe each graduation represents

just 1 unit. Incorrect insulin dosage may occur in patients with poor eyesight, particularly if they are unaware of just how bad their eyesight is. The use of magnifying glasses which clip on to the barrel of the syringe or 'click-count' or blocked syringes can help patients with a visual handicap.

4. **Poor injection technique**: if the same limited area of skin is used repeatedly for injections the subcutaneous tissue may become hard and indurated. Insulin absorption from such areas is sometimes irregular and unpredictable. Occasionally patients may be injecting intradermally instead of subcutaneously.

5. **Poor compliance** is probably the commonest cause of unstable diabetes, but should not be assumed until other possible causes have been excluded. The reasons why regular meal and snack times are essential and why extra food or less insulin is required before exercise should be explained. Dietary errors are sometimes unintentional or inadvertent and a dietary reassessment may be helpful.

Management of unstable diabetes

1. Look for possible causes. This should always include an examination of the injection sites and observation of the patient's technique for drawing up and giving the insulin injection.
2. Adjust insulin dosage to minimise hypoglycaemia.
3. Review the treatment of hypoglycaemia, because overtreatment inevitably causes subsequent hyperglycaemia.

▋ Brittle diabetes

The term 'brittle diabetes' is sometimes used incorrectly to describe any form of unstable diabetes. It should be specifically reserved for those cases where the patient's life is constantly disrupted by severe, and often life-threatening, episodes of hypoglycaemia or hyperglycaemia or both. Defined in this way it is fortunately rare. The aetiology is unknown. Most patients are teenage girls or young women. There is often a history of emotional disturbance or social deprivation. Insulin resistance may occur and makes management even more difficult. Such patients should be managed by the hospital diabetic clinic.

▋ Moderate sustained hyperglycaemia

The management of patients who fail to achieve adequate glycaemic control on their current therapy will be discussed in this section. Definitions of acceptable measures of control are given in Chapter 6, but the diagnosis of sustained hyperglycaemia must be confirmed by laboratory tests, preferably glycosylated haemogobin: results of home blood glucose monitoring and urinalyses alone may be suggestive, but DO NOT confirm the diagnosis.

The poorly-controlled patient on dietary therapy alone clearly requires additional treatment, though a further discussion with the dietitian may be beneficial for the obese patient who is failing to lose weight. The further management of such patients is discussed in Chapter 4 and 5.

Patients on oral hypoglycaemic drugs

Patients on maximum doses of oral hypoglycaemics (OHGs) with poor control usually require insulin therapy, though this may not be practical or necessary in all cases. Three main types of patient are recognised.

1. *Obese, middle-aged patients*
   Such patients form the majority of cases included under this category. They are frequently free from symptoms, but laboratory testing repeatedly confirms high blood glucose and glycosylated haemoglobin readings. As they have insulin resistance, they do not respond to conventional insulin doses and large doses which stimulate the appetite and compound the problem of obesity may be needed. The following approach to such patients is recommended.

   i.   explanation of the need to achieve better control and that insulin may well be needed
   ii.   arrange for review of diet in the hope of achieving better compliance with consequent weight reduction and improved control on OHGs
   iii. frequent review to encourage compliance

   If this fails to achieve improved control with weight reduction then:

   iv.   start on once-daily Ultralente insulin at a low dose (12–16 units/ day), and instruct patients in HBGM (Chapters 5 and 6)
   v.   frequent review with insulin adjustments until acceptable control is achieved.

2. *Symptomatic patients*
   This includes patients who have hyperglycaemic symptoms despite maximum doses of OHGs: often they are not obese. They should be reviewed by the dietitian and then changed to insulin therapy (Chapter 5), with alterations to dosage according to results. It must be remembered that pancreatic carcinoma is more common in diabetic patients,

and the patient who continues to lose weight despite satisfactory control may require further investigation.

3. *Elderly patients*

Old age should not be considered a contraindication to insulin therapy if symptoms persist on OHGs. Moreover, some patients with very high blood glucose readings may deny feeling unwell, and it may only be after the institution of insulin therapy that they realise how symptomatic they previously were. Symptoms such as fatigue, lethargy and weakness that can be caused by chronic hyperglycaemia may have been attributed to old age. Thus these patients require a careful assessment, together with laboratory tests: some may safely tolerate high blood glucose levels, whereas other patients, especially those on multiple-drug therapies, should be transferred to insulin to improve well-being and to reduce the risk of hyperosmolar non-ketotic hyperglycaemic episodes.

Patients on insulin

Patients who continually have high laboratory blood glucose and glycosylated haemoglobin readings can pose a difficult management problem. Several different causes should be considered.

1. *Unreliable home monitoring*

Any insulin treated patient using urinalysis with repeated negative readings should be instructed in HBGM: a high renal threshold for glucose might explain high laboratory results. Insulin doses can then be adjusted if HBGM demonstrates high readings. The combination of relatively normal HBGM readings with high laboratory results may be explained by poor technique or the fabrication of blood glucose readings. The technique of HBGM should be checked to exclude the former: the patient may, for example, be reading the results of the blood glucose immediately after wiping the blood off the stick rather than waiting for the prescribed time.

2. *Poor injection technique*

As explained above, the repeated use of areas of lipohypertrophy may lead to poor absorption and consequent hyperglycaemia. Techniques of drawing up and injection of insulin should be checked.

3. *The dawn phenomenon*

It is recognised that insulin requirements increase in the few hours before waking: persistently high fasting blood glucose results may be caused by relative insulinopenia. If the patient is taking twice-daily soluble and Isophane insulins, it may be advisable to move the second Isophane injection to bedtime to ensure adequate insulin levels in the early morning. Patients on a Novopen and Ultralente regimen should be advised to check a 3 a.m. blood glucose reading to exclude nocturnal hypoglycaemia before increasing the Ultralente dose to correct morning hyperglycaemia.

4. *Other illnesses/medications*
The development of other organic diseases (for example, thyroid disease which is more common in diabetic patients) may be associated with persistent hyperglycaemia. A careful drug history should also be taken.

The management of moderate sustained hyperglycaemia involves the exclusion of common causes and the adjustment of insulin doses as outlined in the section on unstable diabetes.

16 PRACTICAL MANAGEMENT OF TYPE II DIABETES – A SYNOPSIS

This chapter is intended as an *aide-mémoire* to be used in the surgery when seeing a new patient or when carrying out the annual review on a patient with Type II diabetes. A list of equipment and other items needed for this purpose is given in Table 1.

TABLE 1 NECESSARY EQUIPMENT AND OTHER ITEMS

1. Weighing scales
2. Urine test strips for glucose, ketones, protein
3. Stethoscope and sphygmomanometer
4. Snellen chart and pinhole for visual acuity
   Tropicamide 0.5% eye drops (patients with
      dark brown irises may need 1.0%)
   Ophthalmoscope
5. Patellar hammer, C° 128 tuning fork, cotton wool or
      tissue and blunt/sharp pin
6. Venesection equipment
7. Literature, Forms, Certificates, e.g.
      i. Educational and explanatory literature —
         see Appendix 5
      ii. Diabetic identity card for those on oral
         hypoglycaemics — available from BDA
      iii. Urine test records books
      iv. Exemption from prescription charges
         certificates

▉ Initial assessment of a new patient

1. *Confirm the diagnosis*

See Chapter 3 for diagnostic criteria.

2. *Look for evidence of diabetic complications, secondary causes of diabetes and other disease*

See Checklist (Table 2) for history and clinical examination.

3. *Test the urine*

● For protein — if positive arrange MSU to exclude infection
● For ketones — if positive consider whether this is Type I diabetes — see Chapter 3.

TABLE 2 CHECKLIST FOR HISTORY AND EXAMINATION

History	polydipsia, polyuria, weight loss, boils
	pruritus vulvae/balanitis
	burning/tingling/numbness in feet
	cramps/restless legs, claudication
	visual disturbance
	angina, dyspnoea, oedema
	abdominal pain, indigestion
	past history, family history
	drug therapy
Examination	
	blood pressure, heart failure
	epigastric mass, hepatomegaly
	feet — pulses, sensation, ankle jerks, infection, corns, deformity of bones or nails
	eyes — corneal arcus, cataracts, fundi (dilate pupils)
	weight⎫ calculate average weight
	height⎭ for height and age (Appendix 1)

4. *Take blood*

- For glucose — for laboratory confirmation of diagnosis
- For renal function — (creatinine, urea and electrolytes)
- For liver function — if contemplating treatment with metformin

Initial management of a new patient

1. *Explain the diagnosis and reassure the patient*

2. *Give basic dietary advice*

e.g. *Food and Diabetes — just a beginning,* available from BDA.

3. *Arrange for more detailed and specific dietary advice*

See p. 21, The diet prescription. Set a target weight for obese patients — e.g. the average weight for height and age (Appendix 1), but if this seems over-optimistic then compromise.

4. *Consider whether an oral hypoglycaemic (OHG) is indicated*

See Chapter 5. In general an OHG is only indicated at the time of diagnosis if symptoms are very severe or if there are other reasons for wishing to achieve rapid control of hyperglycaemia, e.g. an impending surgical operation. If the diabetes can be controlled by diet alone it helps to emphasise the importance of diet to the patient. If an OHG is prescribed, metformin is usually preferable for the obese patient, because of its anorectic action. If a sulphonylurea is prescribed, teach the patient about hypoglycaemia (Chapter 7).

5. *Review any previous drug therapy*

Could it be relevant to the diabetes? (See Chapter 13.)

6. *Teach urine testing*

The technique should be demonstrated by the practice nurse (see Chapter 6).

7. *Give advice about driving*

i.   Inform DVLC (statutory obligation) and motor insurance company (policy may be invalid if diabetes not declared).
ii. Never drink and drive.
iii. Never drive on an empty stomach if taking a sulphonylurea.

8. *Stop smoking*

Smoking means additional risk for vascular disease.

9. *Other educational advice*

For example on foot care, may be given at this visit if necessary, but is usually best deferred, so as not to swamp the patient with too much information.

10. *Consider referral*

If appropriate consider referral to:

● Dietitian
● Chiropodist
● Ophthalmologist
● District Diabetic Nurse Specialist Service

11. *Provide any necessary literature*

● Dietary advice and other educational literature
● Diabetic identity cards — this incorporates a membership application form for the BDA
● Exemption certificate for prescriptions
● Prescription for urine test strips and medicines

12. *Treat any concomitant disease*

13. *Has the patient any questions?*

14. *Arrange follow-up appointment*

■ First follow-up visit

The timing of the first follow-up visit will usually depend on the severity of symptoms and the degree of hyperglycaemia. An overweight, asymptomatic patient may not need to be seen for 6–8 weeks, whereas a patient with weight loss, thirst and polyuria may need review after 1–2 weeks to ensure that the treatment is starting to take effect.

1. *Are symptoms and hyperglycaemia improving?*

Yes
Continue existing treatment: if obese and target weight has been achieved change to a maintenance diet.

No
Is the patient following his diet (Chapter 4 p.26)? Is an oral hypoglycaemic indicated (Chapter 5)?

2. *Review results of investigations ordered at first visit*

3. *Review any concomitant disease*

4. *Complete the diabetic education*

(See Chapter 9).

5. *Has the patient any questions?*

6. *Arrange next visit*

■ Later follow-up visits

1. *Consider taking a fasting blood sample*

For blood glucose and serum lipid analysis.

2. *Is glycaemic control satisfactory?*

See Chapter 6 for criteria of acceptable control.

Yes

Can calorie restriction be relaxed? Does the dose of oral hypoglycaemic need reducing?

No

- Is the patient following his diet (Chapter 4 p. 26)?
- Does the patient need to start an oral hypoglycaemic or take an increased dose if already on one?
- Is there some other reason for unsatisfactory control, e.g. infection or other illness or stress?

3. *Review any concomitant illness*

4. *Has the patient any questions?*

5. *Arrange next visit*

■ The annual review

The aims of the annual review are to:

1. Ensure the maintenance of satisfactory diabetic control
2. Prevent complications or to detect them at an early stage where intervention may prevent their progression

An appropriate procedure might be as follows:

1. *Enquire*

Enquire about symptoms (see Table 2) and inspect home monitoring record book.

2. *Examine*

Weight — noting any change since last visit
Urine — glucose, protein
Blood pressure — lying and standing
Eyes — visual acuity and fundi
Feet — deformity, corns and callus, pulses, ankle jerks and sensation (see also Chapter 8 Table 5)
Other systems — as appropriate

3. *Take sample*

- For **glucose and glycosylated haemoglobin**
- For **renal function**
- For **serum lipids** if not previously checked, or if previous results abnormal or if weight has increased

4. *Management*

Adjust diet or drug therapy if necessary
Reinforce education, e.g. foot care advice if foot problems have been detected
Consider referral, if necessary, to:

- chiropodist
- dietitian
- diabetes nurse specialist
- ophthalmologist
- hospital diabetic clinic

5. *Has the patient any questions?*

6. *Arrange next visit*

APPENDIX 1

Average weight for height and age

Males

Height metre	ft/in	Age (y) 15–16 kg	lb	17–19 kg	lb	20–24 kg	lb	25–29 kg	lb	30–39 kg	lb	40–49 kg	lb	50–59 kg	lb	60–69 kg	lb
1.52	5.0	44.5	98	51.3	113	55.3	122	58.1	128	59.4	131	60.8	134	61.7	136	60.3	133
1.55	5.1	46.3	102	52.6	116	56.7	125	59.4	131	60.8	134	62.7	137	63	139	61.7	136
1.58	5.2	48.5	107	54	119	58.1	128	60.8	134	62.1	137	63.5	140	64.4	142	63	139
1.60	5.3	50.8	112	55.8	123	59.9	132	62.6	138	64	141	65.3	144	65.8	145	64.4	142
1.63	5.4	53.1	117	57.6	127	61.7	136	64	141	65.8	145	67.1	148	67.6	149	66.2	146
1.65	5.5	55.3	122	59.4	131	63	139	65.3	144	67.6	149	68.9	152	69.4	153	68	150
1.68	5.6	57.6	127	61.2	135	64.4	142	67.1	148	69.4	153	70.8	156	71.2	157	69.9	154
1.70	5.7	59.9	132	63	139	65.8	145	68.5	151	71.2	157	73	161	73.5	162	72.1	159
1.73	5.8	62.1	137	64.9	143	67.6	149	70.3	155	73	161	74.8	165	75.3	166	73.9	163
1.75	5.9	64.4	142	66.7	147	69.4	153	72.1	159	74.8	165	76.7	169	77.1	170	76.2	168
1.78	5.10	66.2	146	68.5	151	71.2	157	73.9	163	77.1	170	78.9	174	79.4	175	78.5	173
1.80	5.11	68.0	150	70.3	155	73	161	75.8	167	78.9	174	80.8	178	81.6	180	80.5	178
1.83	6.0	69.9	154	72.6	160	75.3	166	78	172	81.2	179	83	183	83.9	185	83	183
1.85	6.1	72.1	159	74.4	164	77.1	170	80.3	177	83	183	84.8	187	85.7	189	85.3	188
1.88	6.2	74.4	164	76.2	168	78.9	174	82.6	182	85.3	188	87.1	192	88	194	87.5	193
1.91	6.3	76.9	169	78	172	80.8	178	84.4	186	87.5	193	89.4	197	90.3	199	89.8	198

Weight

Females

Weight

| Age (y) | | 15–16 | | 17–19 | | 20–24 | | 25–29 | | 30–39 | | 40–49 | | 50–59 | | 60–69 | |
| Height | | | | | | | | | | | | | | | | | |
metre	ft/in	kg	lb	kg	lb	kg	lb	kg	lb	kg	lb	kg	lb	kg	lb	kg	lb
1.47	4.10	44	97	44.9	99	46.3	102	48.5	107	52.2	115	55.3	122	56.7	125	57.6	127
1.50	4.11	45.5	100	46.3	102	47.6	105	49.9	110	53.1	117	56.2	124	57.6	127	58.5	129
1.52	5.00	46.7	103	47.6	105	49	108	51.3	113	54.4	120	57.6	127	59	130	59.4	131
1.55	5.1	48.5	107	49.4	109	50.8	112	52.6	116	55.8	123	59	130	60.3	133	60.8	134
1.58	5.2	50.3	111	51.3	113	52.2	115	54	119	57.2	126	60.3	133	61.7	136	62.1	137
1.60	5.3	51.7	114	52.6	116	53.5	118	55.3	122	58.5	129	61.7	136	63.5	140	64	141
1.63	5.4	53.1	117	54.4	120	54.9	121	56.7	125	59.9	132	63.5	140	65.3	144	65.8	145
1.65	5.5	54.9	121	56.2	124	56.7	125	58.5	129	61.1	135	64.8	143	67	148	67.6	149
1.68	5.6	56.1	125	57.6	127	58.5	129	60.3	133	63	139	66.7	147	68.9	152	69.4	153
1.70	5.7	58.1	128	59	130	59.9	132	61.7	136	64.4	142	68.5	151	70.8	156	71.2	157
1.73	5.8	59.9	132	60.8	134	61.7	136	63.5	140	66.2	146	70.3	155	72.6	160	73	161
1.75	5.9	61.7	136	62.5	138	63.5	140	65.3	144	68	150	72.1	159	74.4	164	74.8	165
1.78	5.10	–	–	64.4	142	65.3	144	67.1	148	69.9	154	74.4	164	76.7	169	–	–
1.80	5.11	–	–	66.7	147	67.6	149	69.4	153	72.1	159	76.7	169	78.9	174	–	–
1.83	6.0	–	–	68.9	152	69.9	154	71.7	158	74.4	164	78.9	174	81.6	180	–	–

N.B. Height in shoes and weight in light indoor clothing. The ideal weight for older adults is that appropriate to their heights in the 20–24 year age band.

These tables are reproduced with permission, from Diem, K. and Lentner, C. (Eds) Geigy Scientific Tables (7th edn), Ciba-Geigy, Basle, 1970, p. 711.

APPENDIX 2

■ Diet during intercurrent illness

The following foods each contain approximately 20 grams (2 portions) of carbohydrate:

- 200 ml ($\frac{1}{3}$ pint) of pure fruit juice or Coca Cola (**not** diet coke)
- 200 ml ($\frac{1}{3}$ pint) of milk plus 2 teaspoons of malted milk powder, e.g. Horlicks, Ovaltine
- 2 small blocks of ice-cream
- 2 natural yoghurts or 1 fruit yoghurt
- 2 jelly cubes or 4 large tablespoons of made-up jelly
- 2 bananas or 2 apples or 2 pears or 2 oranges
- 4 teaspoons of sugar

Soups are often suitable but the carbohydrate content of different soups can vary considerably — refer to data in *Countdown* published by the BDA.

Use this information in conjunction with the advice given on pages 25 and 126–127.

APPENDIX 3

■ **Drugs which may affect glycaemic control**

Drugs which are *shown in italics* are of special clinical importance, either because they have a marked effect on glycaemic control (e.g. glucocorticoids) or because they are frequently prescribed (e.g. thiazides).

Some of the more important drug effects are described in Chapter 13.

Drugs which may cause impaired glucose tolerance

Glucocorticoids and ACTH, Oral contraceptives, Danazol, *Thiazides, Chlorthalidone, Diazoxide,* Phenytoin, Salbutamol, Isoniazid, Pentamidine, Asparaginase

Drugs which can potentiate sulphonylureas

Metformin, Phenylbutazone, Azapropazone, Clofibrate, Bezafibrate, MAOIs, Probenecid, *Sulphonamides,* Chloramphenicol, Miconazole, Non-selective beta-blockers

Drugs which can reduce the effect of sulphonylureas

Alcohol — chronic heavy intake, *Rifampicin*

Drugs which can modify symptoms of hypoglycaemia

Alcohol, Beta-blockers, Clonidine

Drugs which contain glucose

Many linctuses, cough lozenges, etc.

APPENDIX 4

▉ Items prescribable on FP10 prescriptions

- Insulins and Oral Hypoglycaemic Drugs
- Syringes: glass 1 ml and 0.5 ml
    'click/count' or 'pre-set' syringes
    for the visually handicapped
    plastic with integral needle 1 ml and 0.5 ml
- Re-usable metal hypodermic needles (26 gauge $\times$ $\frac{1}{2}''$)
- Industrial methylated spirit (70%) } for use in syringe carrying
- Cotton wool } case and for sterilising bung on insulin vial
- Blood glucose test reagent strips: BM 1–44, Dextrostix, Visidex, Glucostix
- Urine test reagent strips: Diastix, Diabur 5000, Clinistix, Ketostix
- Portable spirit-proof carrying case for glass syringes
- Disposable lancets for finger-pricking: Autolet, Monoject
- Needle clipper — for removing needles from disposable syringes

NB: ALL diabetic patients, except those treated by diet alone, are
entitled to an **exemption certificate** for NHS prescriptions.

APPENDIX 5

■ **Useful addresses**

1. Ames Division, Miles Laboratories Ltd
   PO Box 37,
   Stoke Court, Stoke Poges,
   Slough, SL2 4LY

   Glucometer (blood glucose meter)
   Educational literature

2. Becton Dickinson UK Ltd
   Between Towns Road,
   Cowley, Oxford, OX4 3LY

   Educational literature

3. Boehringer Corporation Ltd (BCL)
   Boehringer Mannheim House,
   Bell Lane, Lewes, E. Sussex,
   BN7 1LG

   Reflolux and Reflocheck (blood glucose meters)
   Educational literature

4. British Diabetic Association
   10 Queen Anne Street,
   London,
   W1M 0BD

   Educational literature
   Information packs
   Videos
   Advice on all aspects of diabetes

5. C.P. Pharmaceuticals
   Red Willow Road,
   Wrexham Industrial Estate,
   Wrexham, Clwyd,
   LL13 9PX

   Educational literature

6. Eli Lilly & Co. Ltd
   Dextra Court, Chapel Hill,
   Basingstoke, Hampshire,
   RG21 2SY

   Educational literature

7. English National Board   Course 928 for
    170 Tottenham Court Road,   Diabetes Nursing
    London W1

8. E.M. Products   Identity bracelets
    PO Box 148,
    Edgware, HA8 8JA

9. Golden Key Company   Identity bracelets
    1 Hare Street,
    Sheerness, Kent

10. Hypoguard Ltd   Hypocount blood glucose
    Dock Lane, Melton,   meter
    Woodbridge, Suffolk,
    IP12 1PE

11. Lipha Pharmaceuticals Ltd   Educational literature
    Harrier House, West Drayton,   Videos
    Middlesex, UB7 7QG   Diabetic record cards

12. Medic-Alert Foundation   Identity bracelets and neck-
    17 Bridge Wharf,   laces
    156 Caledonian Road,
    London N1 9UU

13. Medistron Ltd   Glucochek (blood glucose
    6 Lawson Hunt Industrial   meter)
    Park,
    Broadbridge Heath,
    Horsham, W. Sussex,
    RH12 3JR

14. Nordisk UK   Educational literature
    Nordisk House,
    Garland Court,
    Garland Road,
    East Grinstead,
    W. Sussex, RH19 1DN

15. Novo Laboratories Ltd   Educational literature
    Ringway House, Bell Road,
    Daneshill East, Basingstoke,
    Hampshire, RG24 0DN

16. Owen Mumford   Autolet finger prick device
    Brook Hill, Woodstock,
    Oxfordshire, OX7 1TU

17.	Bar Knight Precision Engineering Ltd *5th Floor, 8 Elliott Place, Clydeway Industrial Centre, Glasgow, G3 8EP*	Syringe injector gun (for those who insist on buying one)
18.	Practical Diabetes *The Newbourne Group, Home & Law Publishing Ltd. Greater London House, Hampstead Road, London, NW1 7QQ*	Practical journal on diabetes available free to all health service professionals
19.	Royal College of Nursing *20 Cavendish Square, London, W1M 0AB*	Practice Nurse forum Diabetes Nurse forum Information Packs
20.	Royal College of General Practitioners *14 Princes Gate, Hyde Park, London, SW7 1PU*	Diabetes information package
21.	Royal National Institute for the Blind *224 Great Portland Street, London, W1*	Aids and advice for the visually handicapped
22.	Servier Laboratories Ltd *Fulmer Hall, Windmill Road, Fulmer, Slough, SL3 6HH*	Mini-clinic package for doctors Educational literature Videos
23.	SOS/Talisman Co. Ltd *21 Grays Corner, Ley Street, Ilford, Essex, IG2 7RQ*	Identity bracelets and neck-laces
24.	Ulverston Books *The Green, Bradgate Road, Ansley, Leicester, LE7 7FW*	Large type books for the visually handicapped

INDEX